The
Bumble Bee
Miracle

The
Bumble Bee
Miracle

A Story of Survival from
Inflammatory Breast Cancer

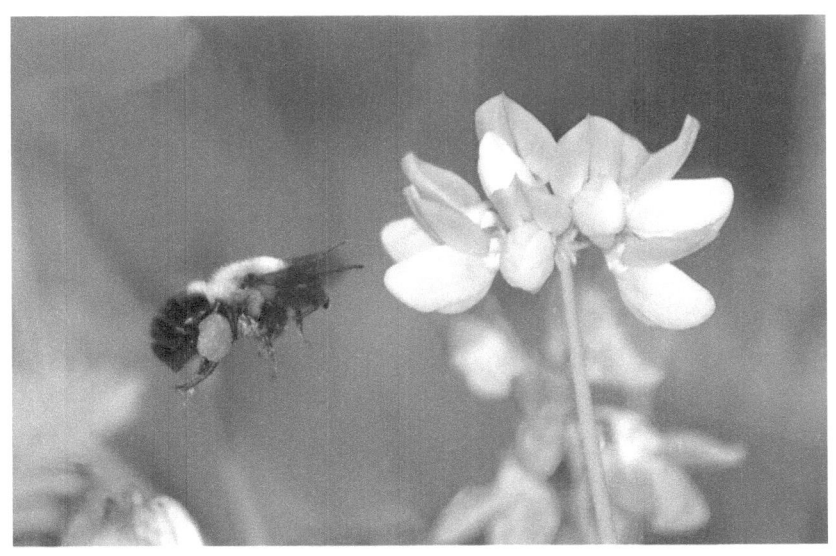

Nina H. Anderson

Library of Congress Control Number: 2007907782
ISBN: Hardcover   978-1-4257-8681-6
                  Softcover   978-1-4257-8675-5

This book was printed in the United States of America.

To order additional copies of this book, contact:
Xlibris Corporation
1-888-795-4274
www.Xlibris.com
Orders@Xlibris.com

43205

CONTENTS

Dedicated to:

Richard, my dear husband of forty-two years, who was constantly by my side. He is a courageous and devoted husband and father . . . .

Shelly, my precious and beautiful daughter, whose courage in the face of trials is an inspiration to me . . . .

And to the loving memory of my oldest daughter, Lynn. I do not know why I am still here and why her life on earth was cut so short, but I know someone who does . . . .

To God be the glory, Great things he hath done!!

ACKNOWLEDGMENTS

I would like to give special thanks to my wonderful and dear oncologist, Dr. Janice Gallashaw with Georgia Cancer Specialist in Atlanta. Her expert knowledge, along with her constant attention and encouragement helped me through the eleven long months of treatment. She helped save my life and she is my hero!

Also, special thanks to my wonderful and dear surgeon, Dr. Elizabeth Steinhaus with Breast Care Specialist in Atlanta. Her astute observations during my first visit led to my early diagnosis and eventual cure. She helped save my life and she too, is my hero!

Special acknowledgment goes to Dr. Gallashaw's Physician Assistant, Kim Sobolick. Her willingness to take as much time as necessary to fully explain any situation was invaluable to me.

Special thanks to the radiologists, nurses, technicians and counselors who devote their time to care for and comfort patients who are in life or death struggles. God bless all of them.

I wish to acknowledge and give special thanks to Dr. C. David Jones, author and retired United Methodist minister, and his lovely wife Barbara for their prayers, guidance, counseling and encouragement to me during my illness and during the writing of this book. What a blessing they have been in my life!

And last, but no least, I wish to thank all of my family, friends and prayer warriors who so lovingly supported me during my battle with Inflammatory Breast Cancer. I pray God's special blessings on each one for every act of kindness and for every prayer lifted on my behalf. Your prayers have been answered! You are my heroes, too!

CHAPTER ONE

THE MONTH OF APRIL

RARE ENCOUNTERS OF THE INTIMATE KIND

You know how when you get past fifty years old, those intimate moments with your spouse are few and far between? Well that's kind of how it was with us. But it was one of those rare evenings when things just seemed to fall in place and it happened! Afterwards my husband, Richard, said that something wasn't right with my right breast. I told him that I had already noticed it and that I thought I might have mastitis. He had no idea what that was, so I explained that it was an infection of the mammary glands which you can sometimes have when you are breastfeeding. I had some redness and swelling and the breast had felt kind of feverish for about a week or two. I told him I guess I would have to make an appointment with my gynecologist and get some antibiotics. It was kind of aggravating to be going through menopause and have to deal with a breast infection. I promised that as much as I hated going to the doctor, I would make an appointment the next day.

When I woke up the next morning, the breast was so swollen that the nipple had inverted. I remembered when I was breast feeding that this same thing had happened when it was feeding time. The breasts would fill with milk and the right nipple would become an "inny" instead of an "outy". I would have to use a nipple shield in order for the baby to be able to nurse. So an inverted nipple with swelling was normal for me. I thought for certain that this was mastitis. I called to get an appointment with my gynecologist and, much to my disappointment, she was not practicing at this time because she had decided to stay home with her children. This was the fourth gynecologist I had had in the past four years. The last three were women and it was just my luck that every time I was ready for my next annual check up, I was informed that they were staying home with their children. I usually liked to go to a female gynecologist because I felt like a woman could understand my problems. Fortunately this time I was seeing someone who was part of a group of gynecologists so I just told the receptionist to pick one for me because I was having some problems and I needed to see someone soon. She said she would call me back to arrange the appointment.

In the meantime, I looked at my calendar and realized it was almost time for my annual mammogram, so I decided that I would try to schedule that appointment as well, especially since it usually takes about two or three weeks to get in. So I called the imaging center where I usually go to have my mammogram to see when I could come in for an appointment. The receptionist said she had an appointment open the very next day. I said, "I'll take it!" I explained to her that I thought I was having a problem. She requested that I call my gynecologist (which of course I did not know who that would be at this time) and request an order for a "diagnostic mammogram". She said to tell them to fax it to them so they would be able to do a more extensive mammogram when I came in the next day. So I called the gynecologist group's office and discovered I had been assigned a new doctor and I asked if it would be possible for them to fax a request for the diagnostic mammogram and of course they were able to do this. My appointment with the gynecologist would be in July. This was April 4th.

So on April 5[th,] 2002, at 2:00 PM I went to have my annual mammogram at the same place I had been going for the past five years. The technician was very nice and she had gotten the fax of the order for the diagnostic tests. I went through the usual eye popping experience only this time it seemed a little more uncomfortable. I waited for the nurse to come back to tell me if the images were OK before getting dressed. When she came in, she said that the radiologist would like to see me. As I was getting dressed, I was thinking that I didn't remember this ever happening before. Maybe they have changed the procedure. When I walked into the slightly darkened room, the radiologist had several x-rays on a lighted background. He began to focus in on an area on my right breast that he said was positioned at about 5 o'clock that indicated there might be a problem. He talked about two types of problems, non-malignant and malignant. I don't remember everything that was said but I do remember the part where he said that he thought that I had a malignant tumor and that the survival rate dropped depending on the size of the tumor. I asked him to explain what he meant. He said with 1 centimeter it is about 90% survival, 1.5 it drops to 80% and so on. I wanted to say, "Are you talking to me?" I have mastitis; I don't have malignant breast cancer! You must have the wrong x-rays up there! But I didn't say anything. The radiologist suggested that we try to get a better image with an ultrasound, so the ultrasound technician escorted me to the ultrasound room where once again I undressed. She tried for forty-five minutes to pick up an abnormality but was unsuccessful. I felt certain by now that they had the wrong person and the wrong x-rays. So I got dressed again and the radiologist came in and said that even though the technician could not identify an abnormality that did not matter. He advised me that I should go straight to a surgeon and just skip the biopsy. He said that they could have the last five years of my images ready for me to take with me. He took my hand, looked me straight in the eye and said if there was ever anything he could do for me to please to let him know. I told him that I would.

Everyone in the area behind the counter was very quiet as I waited for them to prepare the packet of my mammograms. They all seemed to be looking at the floor or the ceiling but never at me. When the nurse handed my mammograms to me she gave me a list of three surgeons that I could call. She told me that one of them was her surgeon who had performed her mastectomy. As I walked out of the office I truly felt like I had just been handed a death sentence. I know I must have been in shock, but somehow I drove home, praying all the while that God would be with me and help me as I brushed back the tears so I could see where I was going. I have always been a praying person. Prayer was the only thing that had sustained me when the unthinkable happened. We lost our precious and beautiful sixteen-year-old daughter, Lynn, in an automobile accident in 1984. Now it seemed the unthinkable had happened again, and once again I called on my Heavenly Father, praying that He would somehow bring me calmness and help me keep my sanity as I faced the uncertain days ahead. I still couldn't believe any of this was true. It must be a bad dream and I will wake up soon and find out that I really only have mastitis!

WHAT'S THE NEXT STEP?

I somehow made it home, but when I got there no one was there. Richard had gone out to do some fieldwork related to his contract job with the county. I couldn't get in touch with my daughter, Shelly, right away. She was teaching, so I just left a message for her to call me. When Richard came home, I began to tell him the news as carefully and calmly as I could. He had question after question and I tried to explain what was said as best as I could remember. Finally, he looked at me and said "They have made a mistake! You told me yesterday that you had mastitis!" He was in denial, too.

We spent the rest of the day and most of the next calling people and trying to find out what we should do next. I called my sisters, Ann and Marilyn, to tell them the news and to get them to help me sort out what the next step would be. I let my parents know and then Shelly called me back so I gave her all of the details, too. She said that there must be some kind of mistake and that we should just wait and see what the surgeon has to say.

I called my employer to let them know the situation and to say that I might have to be out of work for a few days until I could get things sorted out. I called my insurance company to see what they recommended. I had to contact my brand new gynecologist and get a referral for a surgeon or specialist in order for my insurance to cover the services. I called my cousin, Glenna, who had just had some breast surgery a short time ago, and asked her if she could recommend someone. Her surgeon was also the same surgeon who had operated on the receptionist at the imaging center and she highly recommended her. By this time it was late in the evening on Friday and I would have to wait until Monday to schedule any appointments. We had a long weekend ahead of us.

We went to our little church, Shiloh United Methodist, on Sunday. I had already called our pastor and some of our church family to let them know and to ask them to please pray for my family and me. They already had me on the prayer list, which was very comforting. I love our little church. It was actually built in 1865. The lumber used in the sanctuary was hand planed by the church members who had built the church. The beautiful stained glass windows, which depict scenes from the Bible are so beautiful. They were added in the early 1950's. We are a small congregation and everyone there always shares each other's joys as well as the sorrows. We are a close-knit group. When our daughter was killed, it was as if each member had suffered the loss of a daughter along with us.

Early on Monday morning I contacted the gynecologist's office and requested the referral from him to see the surgeon whose name kept popping up. It was like confirmation that I should see her. I then called the surgeon's office to schedule an appointment which I thought would probably be a week or two away. I told the receptionist the situation and she said that she had an appointment "in the morning" at 9:30 AM. I said, "I'll take it!" She said to come a little early so we could fill out forms for a new patient. So we got up very early the next morning and planned to leave by 8:00 AM in order to get to Northside Hospital by 9:00 AM. It was only 20 miles away, but it would be during rush hour traffic so we knew it would take about an hour to get there. When we got there I signed in and they gave me all of the paperwork to fill out for a new patient. I had brought my five years of mammograms with me as instructed. When I finished the paperwork and went back to the counter, the nurse said they did not have me listed for an appointment today but they did have me for "Wednesday morning". I told her that I had called the day before and the person had told me there was an opening "in the morning". Apparently, I had misunderstood and heard "in the morning" instead of "Wednesday morning". Richard was with me and we were both so disappointed. We asked if there was any way the surgeon could see me today, but she said it would be impossible today. She said she would give the surgeon my images so that she would have time to review them before I came back tomorrow.

So we drove back home to spend another day and another night waiting to take the next step. We got up bright and early once again and battled the Wednesday morning rush hour traffic. At least I wouldn't have to fill out paperwork this time. We got there a little early and we could tell that the surgeon was already behind with her appointments, so we had quite a wait before I was finally called back. I had to undress from the waist up and put on a special gown. I then had to wait in another waiting room with all the other ladies who had on the same type gown, but some were different colors. I finally figured out that my surgeon's gown color was blue. I think I must have read every magazine there was to read before I was called back to an examination room, where I had to wait once again. Finally the surgeon came in and I told her my story and how I thought I had mastitis, but the radiologist seemed to think it was a malignant tumor and that I should just skip the biopsy and go straight to surgery. She had reviewed my images and said that she really couldn't see much of an image of anything. She examined me and decided that she would do a biopsy against the advice of the radiologist. She said she would never think of performing surgery on someone without first doing a biopsy to see what she was up against.

So we moved from the examination room to another room where the biopsies were performed. I was given some local anesthetic, which was injected into the breast area, especially around the nipple area. She took several biopsies, which included a "core" biopsy and a surgical "skin" biopsy. All the time she kept asking me if I was OK, and I kept saying that I was. I felt something running down the side of my chest and I tried to look at what they were doing, but she quickly told me not to look. I told her I couldn't feel any pain. She said that was good.

Once she finished and the area was bandaged, they gave me an ice pack to place in my bra to keep the swelling and pain down. I was taken back to the examination room. She came in and told me that the biopsy would be sent to a lab and that it would take three to five days to get the results back. She would call me as soon as she got them. So we went back home once again to wait for the next step. This was on Wednesday, April 10th.

We had not heard anything by Friday, so it would be another long weekend of waiting. On Monday, April 15th (Tax Day), I was working at my office in my home as usual. My sister, Ann, had come over to work with me that day. Richard had planned to work at home so he would be there when the call came in. We waited all day trying to stay busy and not think about the big monster in the back of our minds. It was late afternoon when we finally got the call from my surgeon. Richard picked up the extension so he could hear what she had to say. She told us that she had gotten the results back and that it was MALIGNANT! She told me I had INFLAMMATORY BREAST CANCER and that it was INOPERABLE! She said she would refer me to an oncologist who would determine what options might be available and which would be best. We listened to her say all of these things and it was beginning to sink in. I was feeling kind of numb all over and my knees began to shake uncontrollably. We hung up the phone and told Ann what she had said. We all hugged and cried. I was silently praying for calmness and not to panic.

Once we calmed down a bit (my prayers were answered), I told them that we needed to let the rest of the family know, but when we tell them, except for Shelly, that we would not use the word "inoperable", at least not yet. I remember when Richard's Dad was diagnosed with Lung Cancer that he was told that the cancer was inoperable and that he only had about six months to live. So, to me, the word inoperable meant terminal. They agreed that this would be best. My Dad was eighty-five and my Mother was eighty-one, Richard's Mother was in poor health, so I wanted to spare them from worry as much as possible, but I felt that I needed to let Shelly know. We started making calls, but when Richard called his Mother and tried to tell her, he couldn't get the words out and he just handed the phone to Ann. The rest of the day was very hard, very hard indeed.

Even though it was late in the afternoon when we got the call, the surgeon had managed to schedule an appointment for the very next day with an oncologist. She called to give us the name and directions. So we would wait another night to see what the next step would be. During the days ahead I would come to realize that, with God's help, my focus would be "what is the next step?" . . . . one step at a time, one day at a time . . . .

INFLAMMATORY BREAST CANCER (IBC)

Almost everyone that I had ever known who had breast cancer, had a lumpectomy or a mastectomy. Why couldn't I have one of these operations? Was the cancer so far advanced that it was useless to operate? Was I going to die? I had only had the symptoms a few weeks and I never even had any pain, just a little soreness. Surely, surely there has been some kind of mistake! I decided I would go on the Internet and find out what I could about this Inflammatory Breast Cancer.

If you've ever tried to look up a disease on the Internet you will understand when I say that I learned more than I ever wanted to know about Inflammatory Breast Cancer. It is a very rare form of breast cancer, comprising only about 3% of all breast cancers, so there was not a great deal of information out there but what was there was all bad and was way more than I ever wanted to know. The following article written by Dr. Jeff Patton of Tennessee Oncology was taken from the National Breast Cancer Foundation, Inc. website: Breast Cancer Signs & Symptoms—Inflammatory Breast Cancer:

Inflammatory Breast Cancer

Inflammatory breast cancer is a unique and uncommon type of breast cancer. It is unique in that inflammatory breast cancer does not produce a distinct mass or lump that can be felt within the breast. The lack of a lump or mass also makes inflammatory breast cancer difficult to detect by mammograms. Inflammatory breast cancer cells infiltrate the skin and lymph vessels of the breast. When the lymph vessels become blocked by the breast cancer cells the breast typically becomes red, swollen, and warm. The skin changes associated with inflammatory can cause the breast skin to look like the skin of an orange, a finding called peau d'orange. The appearance of the breast is similar to other inflammatory conditions such as cellulitis or mastitis. Other possible associate symptoms include enlarged lymph nodes under the arm or above the collarbone on the affected side.

Inflammatory breast cancer is diagnosed based upon the results of a biopsy and the clinical judgment of the treating physician. Typically, inflammatory breast cancer grows rapidly and requires aggressive treatment. There are two aspects to treating all breast cancer, local treatment and systemic or total body treatment. Because inflammatory breast cancer is aggressive, most oncologists recommend both systemic and local treatment. The typical sequence of treatment is to start with chemotherapy, systemic treatment, followed by surgery and radiation therapy, which are the local treatments, often followed by additional chemotherapy and possibly hormone treatments. With aggressive treatment using this multimodality approach, the 5 year survival for inflammatory breast cancer has improved significantly from an average survival of 18 months to an approximately 50% survival rate at 5 years.

How many cases of IBC are diagnosed each year?

The numbers vary, but approximately 1% to 2% of newly diagnosed invasive breast cancers (that have spread beyond the breast) in the United States are described as inflammatory breast cancers.

What are the symptoms of IBC?

Symptoms may include:

- One breast larger than the other
- Red or pink skin
- Swelling
- Rash (entire breast or small patches)
- Orange-like texture (peau d' orange)
- Skin hot to the touch
- Pain and/or itchiness
- Ridges or thickened areas of breast
- Nipple discharge
- Nipples that appear inverted or flattened
- Swollen lymph nodes under the armpit
- Swollen lymph nodes of the neck (sometimes)

What should people do if they have IBC symptoms?

If one or more symptoms continue for more than a week, look for information and talk to someone who is experienced with this particular type of breast cancer.

How old are typical IBC patients at diagnosis?

The median age range is between 45 and 55 years old, but there may be patients either younger or older. The symptoms must guide the diagnosis, and age should not be used to exclude it.

How well do diagnostic tests work in identifying IBC?

IBC typically **cannot** be identified through:

Mammogram—Because IBC usually does not occur in the form of a lump (the cancer is spread throughout breast tissue), it is difficult to detect with a mammogram. The most characteristic mammography findings consist of swelling of the skin.

Ultrasound—This test confirms the swelling (edema) of the skin and can better identify breast nodules (if present). It also is the most appropriate test for the evaluation of lymph nodes.

Magnetic Resonance Imaging (MRI)—This is probably the most sensitive test because it includes a functional description of the abnormal findings. It should be included among the diagnostic tests once the pathological diagnosis is confirmed. It is extremely useful in evaluating the clinical response to chemotherapy.

Core biopsy—Typically, fine-needle aspiration or a core biopsy (removal of tissue with a needle) is performed to obtain a pathological diagnosis of invasive disease, but these diagnostic procedures are not appropriate for IBC because of the peculiar growth pattern in the breast lymphatic system.

What diagnostic tests identify IBC?

Surgical biopsy—Most of the time a skin biopsy or a surgical biopsy is necessary. These procedures are able to collect larger samples that include the skin and underlying tissue with higher chances to identify the cancer cells.

PET Scan—In the near future, this could be one of the most important diagnostic staging tests for IBC, though it still is under study. We have found that with the PET scan we can see more disease

We can see lymph nodes far from the breast, which tells us we have a metastatic cancer already at the time of diagnosis. If we limit staging to mammogram, CT (computed tomography—computerized X-rays) and bone scans we may miss different components of this inflammatory spreading, which may have significant consequences in the way we treat the cancer and the way we process patients.

What is the survival rate for IBC?

The five-year median survival rate for inflammatory breast cancer is approximately 40%. The main reasons for such a disappointing outcome are multiple and include: a delay in diagnosis, the lack of expertise in treating IBC because it is so rare and the relative resistance the disease has to standard chemotherapeutic agents.

With regard to the first critical issue, it is important to keep in mind that IBC is a fast-growing cancer (it can spread within weeks), and it is often mistaken for something other than breast cancer, such as a rash or infection.

What are common mistakes in treating IBC?

A surgeon might want to remove the breast too early, which would increase the chance of local recurrence (return of the disease).

A radiation oncologist with experience in treating IBC also is important. IBC might require a different schedule than most breast cancers. You might need two treatments a day, instead of one, because this is a highly aggressive tumor. Patients also need a specific chemotherapy dose.

A particular challenge with treating IBC is that it is difficult to measure response since a nodule or mass is usually not present. If patients have had incorrect treatment, it may be hard to go back and improve the prognosis (outcome).

How is IBC currently treated?

We typically treat IBC with chemotherapy before surgery, and we also are using drugs like Herceptin® (trastuzumab) or Tykerb™ (lapatinib) in a subset of IBC patients who have the HER-2 gene. One of our challenges is to improve our current treatments. We are focused on finding ways to eliminate microscopic disease to prolong survival. [1]

THE WHIRLWIND TOUR!

On April 16, 2002, I was scheduled to see an oncologist, which is a specialist in the treatment of malignant cancer. Hopefully we would find out what would be the next step. When my name was called, I was ushered into an examining room and was asked to undress from the waist up and put a paper gown with the opening in the front. The physician's assistant examined me and we talked about my symptoms and what had happened up until now. When the doctor came in we talked some more. I asked him if he thought that I could be cured. His answer was that every person was different and that it was absolutely possible that I could achieve good health again. For the first time since I heard the words malignant cancer, I had a ray of hope. He reviewed my file and recommended that I should have four chemotherapy treatments consisting of two drugs called Adriamycin and Cytoxan (A/C Treatments). The treatments would be given in three-week intervals in order to have time to recuperate from each treatment. After completing these treatments, he recommended that I have a mastectomy and possibly more chemotherapy and radiation after the surgery.

Because of the aggressiveness of the cancer, the oncologist said that I would need to begin the chemotherapy treatments as soon as possible. In order for that to happen, I would need a battery of tests just to determine if I would be able to withstand the treatment that was being prescribed. It was already Tuesday afternoon and he wanted me to start the A/C treatments on Friday! I would have to have a Brain CT Scan, a Bone CT Scan, a Whole Body CT Scan and an Echo Cardiogram.

The person who arranges the scheduling began making calls and, by some kind of miracle, I was scheduled for all of these tests on Wednesday and Thursday. The results had to be back to my oncologist before 11:00 AM on Friday, which was when they were able to schedule my appointment for my first chemotherapy treatment! He would have to know by then if it was going to be possible for me to take the treatments. We were given specific instructions on where and when to go for all of these tests. I felt like I was in a whirlwind and my head was spinning from trying to absorb all that was taking place. Thank goodness Richard and Shelly were there with me to help listen to all that was said.

During the next two days I was like a robot, going from one imaging center to another. We had completed all tests scheduled for Wednesday, so I only had one more test on Thursday which was a Whole Body CT Scan. Because I am allergic to Iodine, which is what they use in the IV when you have a Whole Body CT Scan, I had to be pre-medicated so I would not have a reaction. We had managed to get the prescription on Wednesday for the pre-medication for the test, which was scheduled for Thursday. I had to take the medication the night before and also thirty minutes before the test. When my daughter and I got to the imaging center on Thursday for this last test, we were told that someone had made a mistake. Since I was allergic to the dye, I would have to be admitted as an outpatient in the hospital so that if anything happened during the test I would be where I needed to be. That was not a comforting thing to hear and besides, I had to have this test done TODAY. I couldn't wait until tomorrow because there wouldn't be enough time to get the results before my treatment, which was scheduled for Friday. They hurriedly called the hospital and they told us if we could get to the hospital within thirty minutes they could take me that day. Thankfully we were only a few blocks from the hospital, so we ran to the parking lot and drove as fast as we could to get to the hospital.

It is a huge hospital so we were hoping we would find the right place that we were supposed to be. When we got there, I had to go through admissions and also my insurance company had to be notified that I was being admitted so they could pre-approve the procedure. Somehow we got all of the necessary paperwork and processing completed and we were sent to the waiting room to wait for my name to be called to have the test. We only had to wait about an hour but it seemed like a lot longer. I tried not to think about what might happen if I had a reaction! I just turned it over to the Lord and put my trust in Him to get me through it. When the test was finally completed, without any problems, I breathed a sigh of relief and said a prayer of thankful praise.

In all of the information that I had received and tried to absorb about chemotherapy, I had learned that with one of the treatments (Adriamycin) you always loose your hair. Not just your hair on your head but every hair on your body, including your eyelashes, eyebrows and everywhere else. The Adriamycin kills the hair follicles. I was advised to try to get a wig before my hair all fell out so that I would be able to match it more closely to my own color. So, on Thursday afternoon, April 18th, before my first chemo (on the way home from the last day of testing), I stopped at a boutique that specialized in items for breast cancer patients. I must have tried on fifteen or twenty different wigs, but none of them really matched or even looked like me, but I was desperate to get this ordeal over with since I did not know how I would feel after the treatments started. So I finally made the decision and I bought a wig that was close to my color and length. The price tag was more than I really wanted to pay (about $300), but at this point I didn't want to shop around. Besides, the salesperson said that my insurance company would pay something toward the purchase. The wig had a hint of auburn in it, which made it a little darker than my own hair. I decided to put it on and wear it to my parent's to see their reaction.

I arrived at my parent's home and began to tell them about all of the tests we had completed during the last two days and how, by some miracle, we were able to work out all the details and get them done before my chemo the next day. We talked for a while and finally I asked them how they liked my hair. They both said it looked fine. I asked if they noticed anything different, but they said no. Well!, I thought, this was great! They didn't even notice it was a wig! When I told them, they just couldn't believe it. So when I left there, I was really feeling good about the wig. What I didn't think of at the time was that my Dad is blind in one eye and can barely see out of the other one and my Mother's eyesight wasn't much better!

When I got home to show Richard, he was not impressed to say the least. He said the color wasn't right and it wasn't my "style". He liked my real hair better. I told him that so did I, but in about 10-14 days it would all be gone. That's right! It only takes 10-14 days for all of your hair to fall out after the first high dose of Adriamycin! I put the wig away until later when I would need it.

DECISIONS, DECISIONS

At some point during all of this testing that was going on, someone had suggested that maybe I should get a second opinion from another oncologist regarding the treatment that should be prescribed. I had a friend who worked for another oncologist group and miracle of miracles she was able to get me an appointment at 8:00 AM on Friday morning. I needed to hear if there were any other options out there for me, but I had already made up my mind that I was going to have my first chemo at 11:00 AM no matter what other options were presented.

We met with the new oncologist who was very thorough. During my consultation with the first oncologist, his assistant performed the examination and he was not even in the room. This time, instead of the assistant, the oncologist examined me, even measuring by touch the size of the tumor, which she estimated was about 5.5 cm! When she told me the size, I immediately remembered what the radiologist had said about survival rate and centimeters, trying to calculate in my head from 1cm—90% survival rate, 1.5 cm 80% survival rate, etc . . . but I quickly put that thought out of my mind. After all, every person is different!

Richard and Shelly had come with me to hear the other options, if any. After the exam, we were ushered into the doctor's office where she presented some very interesting statistics. She talked with us extensively about the treatment and new studies that had been done. She recommended a slightly different approach to the treatment. Her recommendation for treatment was to have four chemotherapy treatments of Adriamycin and Cytoxan at three-week intervals and then four more chemotherapy treatments using Taxotere at three-week intervals and then have surgery. After surgery there would be thirty-five radiation treatments to the chest area. The thing that caught our attention the most was the fact that she said some patients were actually cancer free at the time of surgery after going through the eight up front (neo adjuvant) treatments.

She also informed us that in reviewing my records, which my surgeon had faxed to her, that there were two more tests that she felt needed to be performed. One was called the Her-2-neu test and the other was an ER/PR test. These tests could give more insight as to specific treatments in the future. She said it was imperative that we find out if there was enough tissue left from the original biopsy to allow for these tests to be performed. If not, I would need to have another core biopsy before my chemo at 11:00 AM or the opportunity to get this tissue for the tests may be missed because of destruction of the cancer cells by the chemo. We all began praying that there would be enough tissue, because I didn't think I could go through a consultation and examination, another biopsy and my first chemo all in one day.

I called my current oncologist who was administering the first chemo treatment in less than two hours. I asked him if he could find out if there was enough tissue left to perform these two tests, which were not performed during the initial biopsy. He said he would call the pathologist at the hospital and find out. In the meantime the second oncologist was also working on finding out about the tissue. Apparently the pathologist who could give us the answer would not be in until 10:00AM or later! He would then have to find the sample and call her back. It was about 9:15AM when we left the second oncologist's office.

We had left our cell phone number with both oncologists and just got in the car and drove around waiting to hear from somebody. It was a very tense time for all of us. We were all just praying that everything would work out. Finally, at about 10:35AM the second oncologist called and said that there was enough tissue left to perform the test. What a relief! She advised me to ask my current oncologist to order the Her-2-neu test and the ER/PR test. My current oncologist was calling as I hung up with the second, also telling us that there was enough tissue. I asked him to please order the tests and that I would be there shortly for my first chemo. In the midst of the whirlwind the Lord had answered our prayers! And now, on to the next step! The whirlwind was almost over for this week!

We drove to my oncologist's office and I began to prepare myself inwardly to go through the treatment. Everyone was so very nice and helpful as we were ushered to the area where the treatment would be given. I was informed that I would be prepared for the treatment by first inserting an IV through which the treatment would be administered. I would receive some pre-medication for nausea and to prevent any allergic reaction to the chemo. This would take about thirty minutes. Then a nurse would fill a very large syringe with Adriamycin (known as Big Red), which would be pushed through the IV by a nurse, it would not be a drip. This procedure would take about two hours for the first treatment. They wanted to go very slow in case any reaction developed. After completing the Adriamycin, they would start an IV drip for the Cytoxan, which would take one and one half hours. I just kept thinking about a scripture that I had once read (I couldn't remember the book, chapter or verse) that said if we believed in and trusted God that we would be able to drink poison and it would not hurt us. That's exactly what I would be taking into my body, poison to kill the cancer. I just hoped and prayed that it wouldn't kill me in the process.

Richard and Shelly and my sister, Ann, were there with me in person and so was God's Holy Spirit, the Comforter, bringing me peace and calmness through the whole ordeal. As I sat there in the chair receiving the treatment, I imagined everyone who was praying for me standing in a circle around me and I felt the power of prayer lifting me up and helping me through each minute of the three and one half hours of the treatment. As I lay there in the recliner, I looked outside and I noticed several bumblebees flying outside of this fifth floor window. I remembered reading somewhere that, according to the laws of aerodynamics, bumblebees can't fly! It's impossible! But there they were, leaping over tall buildings, sometimes at the speed of bullets. It suddenly dawned on me that if bumblebees can fly, then anything is possible with God as our Creator! God had used this fuzzy, furry, fat little fellow to remind me of his awesomeness and power.

It was late on Friday afternoon when I completed my first chemotherapy treatment. We decided to stop for a bite to eat on the way home. I was feeling totally exhausted from the week's activities, especially from the treatment. I was able to eat some soup for dinner, but I wasn't feeling very well and I didn't want anything else. Besides, the soup didn't taste right. It was like my taste buds weren't working. I had been given a prescription for a medication (Zofran) that would help to ward of the nausea that would surely come. I was really dreading that part, because for me, throwing up is right before dying. I was to start taking the medication that night and continue to take it for three days. I had to take all of the pills exactly as prescribed in order to prevent the nausea. If I didn't and the nausea set in and I began to throw up, it would be very hard to reverse it. I felt a little nauseous now and then, but never so bad that I had to throw up. I was just praying that the Lord would help me get through it.

We had a long weekend to do a lot of thinking and to try and decide if I would change oncologists and treatment methods. It would mean six months of chemotherapy instead of only three months and then surgery. As I talked about the pros and cons with Richard and Shelly and my other family members, I kept coming back to the statement that the second oncologist had made that some patients were cancer free after the eight neo adjuvant treatments. I was kind of in a daze after all I had experienced in the past two weeks. We managed to go to church on Sunday morning and just doing that gave me a sense of being normal again. I guess being in God's house and feeling the presence of the Holy Spirit and the love and support expressed to me by everyone there was just what I needed.

When I woke up on Monday morning, I lay in bed for a while because I was somewhat anxious about how I would feel. Would I be able to go to work and focus on the tasks at hand? Would I have the energy to continue for the whole day? Would I have to decide to work or not to work? All of these thoughts were racing through my mind. I was praying that God would be with me and help me. Then, suddenly, I looked at my hands and my feet and legs, I felt of my arms and my face and I thought, "I don't feel like I am going to die today, so I might as well get up and get moving and face the day".

Fortunately, my office was downstairs in our basement so I didn't have to worry about getting to work and having to drive back home if I did get sick or something. I had been working in my home for a little over a year, so I had developed a discipline in order to keep responsibilities of home from interfering with my 9 to 5 hours at work. It was my routine to get up and get dressed in casual business clothes and put on my make-up just as if I were going to my old office, which had been located in Buckhead (a business community in north Atlanta). This was my way of getting into a work mode.

Once I finally got up that first Monday morning after my first chemotherapy treatment, I was amazed at how quickly I fell back into my routine, which really proved to be a kind of therapy for me, just to be doing something normal again. The first thing I did when I got downstairs was to make the phone call to my current oncologist's office and tell them of our decision to see another oncologist who had presented a different option of treatment. I requested that they send all of my records to my new oncologist. I thanked them for their care and treatment, but felt that this was what we needed to do. I called the second oncologist's office and they scheduled me for a visit on Wednesday, May 1st, to talk about the treatments and the schedule in more detail and to check my blood counts after the first chemo.

Once I had finished the calls, I started to work. I quickly realized that the responsibilities of my job enabled me to keep my mind off myself, and it left no time for any pity parties. I was able to focus on the task at hand and when I finished something it gave me a feeling of great accomplishment. I praised God for answering my prayer. So this became my routine each morning. I would wake up, assess how I felt and I would say, "Well, I don't think I am going to die today, so I might as well get up and get moving. Hi Ho, Hi Ho, it's off to work we go!

I made it very well through the first few days of working after my first chemo treatment, but I noticed that my energy level would wane about every two hours. Fortunately, since I was working at home, I could go upstairs and rest when I needed to. I learned very quickly that if I were to continue working that I would need to listen to my body and pace myself during the day in order to go the distance. I thanked the Lord for continuing to sustain me each day.

Sometime during those first few days after my first chemo, we remembered that we had reservations at Edgewater Beach Resort in Panama City for a little spring get-a-way. We had made them about six months earlier. The dates were April 24-28. So another decision had to be made. Would we cancel our reservations or should we try to keep to our normal schedule as much as possible. I wasn't thrilled about leaving home so soon after my first chemo and, more importantly, being so far away from my oncologist. What if something happened? What if I started throwing up and couldn't stop? What if I had a delayed reaction to the chemo? All of these fears kept going through my mind. I knew that I probably needed some down time after all that I had been through and so did Richard. He and I both were still trying to squeeze in working at our desk jobs in between all of this and we were both pretty exhausted. I called my oncologist to get her advice on whether we should go or not and she recommended that I should go if I felt like it. So I put my fears aside and we decided to go and try to enjoy a few days at the beach. It would be a time for us to get some rest and to reflect on all that had happened. Besides, my oncologist was only a phone call away.

It was very relaxing at the beach. The usual crowd of people was not there and we could choose our spot at the pool. We enjoy walking the beach in the early morning when very few people are up, so we did that everyday, but I couldn't walk as far as we usually did, I guess because of the chemo. Richard went deep sea fishing one day, so that got his mind off things. I was able to do some reading that day and it helped to get my mind off of my situation, too. Fortunately, I did not have any problems while we were there. My taste buds were still not working very well, but I managed to eat something at each meal. I could tell I was losing some weight (I could stand to loose a few pounds), but I didn't want to be malnourished in addition to having breast cancer, and I needed to keep my strength up for the days ahead.

CHAPTER TWO

THE MONTH OF MAY

A LITTLE GOOD NEWS!

When we returned from our spring get-a-way, it was time to face reality again. We managed to catch up on some of our work, which kept piling up while we were gone. On Wednesday, May 1st, I had an appointment with my oncologist. She had an office only six miles from our house and she was there every Wednesday. This was great because we didn't have to deal with a lot of traffic. We left home fifteen minutes before my appointment and we made it there with time to spare. When my name was called, Richard and I were escorted to an examination room. There the doctor examined me for the second time and gave me some very encouraging news. She said that after only one chemo treatment she could tell that the tumor had already begun to shrink. We were very excited about this good news, especially me! In addition, all of the results from the tests that were performed before my first chemo did not reveal any solid evidence of involvement in any other areas! Praise the Lord! However there were some small spots on my liver that were probably cysts, which she said could have been there since I was born.

We were then escorted to the lab where I had a blood test and, as expected, my white cell count had dropped. An antibiotic was prescribed as a precautionary measure. I was told to stay away from crowds so that I wouldn't "catch" anything while my white cells (the disease fighting cells) were so low. Also, I had been having heartburn and they gave me a prescription for Prilosec. So this prescription, along with the antibiotic were the only two medications I would be taking for now. I was scheduled for another appointment to see the nurse on Friday when another blood count would be performed. If my counts were the same or better, no injections, but if my counts had dropped, I would have to start taking injections that would boost my cell counts. I decided I would wait and find out more about the injections when, and if, I had to take them.

I was also told that I had tested positive for the ER/PR receptor test, which was good. I didn't know exactly why yet, but it was good. However, the Her-2-neu test was not so good. Over expression of the Her-2-neu receptor has been found to correlate with more aggressive forms of cancer. The higher the number of Her-2-neu genes in a cancer cell, the more aggressive the cancer is. Most cancer cells have two Her-2-neu genes per cancer cell. My average count per cancer cell was 15.6! The oncologist said that she had only had one other patient with a higher count. I thought about asking her how the patient was doing, but I decided against it for now.

During the examination, the doctor checked for mouth sores and asked if I had developed a sore throat. I did not have either, which was good. I also still had all my hair, but I didn't know for how long.

After finding out the good news that the tumor was shrinking, the oncologist decided to wait for three months to do another body scan to really have a good comparison and we could also see if there were any changes in the liver spots that had appeared on the first body scan. I had lost a couple of pounds during the first week, but I had managed to gain some back. We had a lot of positive things during this visit and it was very encouraging. I knew that I had a lot of "family, friends and prayer warriors" who were praying for me and I could feel their prayers, and I could feel God's presence every day helping me through this and giving me peace and calmness. I decided I would keep all of them updated by sending out an e-mail as often as I could to let everyone know about my progress and to thank them for their care and concern and especially for their continuing prayers.

HAIR TODAY, GONE TOMORROW

I returned to the oncologist's office on Friday morning, May 3rd, to have another blood test or CBC as they referred to it. My counts were still very low and I was once again reminded not to be around crowds of people and especially small children, who can carry all sorts of germs in their little bodies and nobody even knows it. Today was my Dad's 86th birthday, and we had planned a huge celebration. We invited lots of friends and family from near and far. My four brothers and two sisters were planning on having a fish fry on Friday night, breakfast on Saturday morning, and then a barbeque for lunch. We had planned for about one hundred and twenty five people to be in attendance to the fish fry and barbeque. The breakfast would be for out-of-town guests and anyone who wanted to help prepare for the huge lunch. We were doing all of the preparation and cooking for the events. Fortunately, we had our own barbeque grill and pit that my Georgia Tech Engineer brother, Gene, had elaborately constructed. We planned all of the menus and purchased all of the supplies. I was in charge of salads and desserts, so I had to be there. I continued to take the antibiotics and just prayed that I would not be exposed to anything. I tried not to do too much hugging, but everyone knew about my cancer and they all wanted to come and speak to me and give me a hug. I was so humbled by all of the concern for me and my family. I am sure that a lot of healing took place with each prayerful hug that day.

I wore a hat all day on Friday, because I had noticed a lot of hair in my comb that morning, so I knew the falling out process had started. After the fish fry and clean up that night, we made everything ready for the breakfast the next morning and then we all went home to get some rest. It was a wonderful day of seeing family and friends and celebrating Dad's birthday.

The alarm went off at 6:00 AM on Saturday morning. I reached over and switched on the lamp near the bed. I placed my hand on my pillow to push myself up and that's when I saw it. My pillow was covered with strands of my hair. I touched my head and hair and discovered that it was coming out by the handfuls. I ran to the bathroom mirror and grabbed a brush and starting brushing through my hair. With every brush stroke more hair came out. Finally all I had left were some patches of hair here and there. I woke Richard up to show him what had happened. My sister, Ann, had spent the night with us, so I woke her up to see this phenomenon. I was trying not to cry, but the more I looked in the mirror, the more the urge to cry came creeping up in my throat and into my eyes. The tears began to fall softly as we talked about what I should do. Someone at the chemo treatment center had suggested that when it starts to come out that it is just better to go ahead and use some hair clippers to buzz it all off. I looked at my hair as I held the clippers in my hand. I finally handed the clippers to my sister and said "Just do it!" In less than a minute all of my hair that was left was on the floor. I began to pick it up and to clean out my brush and remove it from my pillow. I put all of it in a plastic zip lock bag. I just wanted to save it for a little while.

My head felt stubbly where the patches had been. I looked like something out of Star Trek. All I needed was the pointed ears! I looked at Richard, who had been quietly standing by. I looked at his balding head, and I apologized for anything I had ever said about his going bald. Now I knew how he felt, although it wasn't exactly the same. He said that, personally, he thought hair was over rated. He was trying to make me feel better. As I sat there looking in the mirror, I thought that it could be worse. Besides, at least my hair would grow back after the chemo was over. Richard was just stuck with his bald head.

We all got ready and started to make plans for the day. I decided to wear a headband and a hat. I just wasn't ready for the wig yet. A group of Shelly's teacher friends at school had given me several hats, headbands, scarves and turbans that had been used by other women who had lost their hair because of breast cancer treatment. I was so amazed at all of the concern, especially from people I didn't even know. I was also very thankful for their thoughtfulness. Since I had worn a hat yesterday, maybe no one would notice any difference at the Saturday festivities.

We had a great time and a great turnout for the Saturday celebration. There was more food than you could imagine. We had all kinds of salads and vegetables and desserts. We had ribs, fried chicken, roasted turkeys, prime rib and hams. Gene had even cooked some cold boiled shrimp to have as an appetizer. I was so thankful that my taste buds had returned so I could at least enjoy the food, even if I didn't have any hair. Dad really enjoyed all of the attention and I could tell he was so proud of all of us for making it all happen.

By the end of the day we were all stuffed and I was totally exhausted. Shelly had come for her grandfather's celebration and to celebrate her birthday which was on May 5th. She would be 29 on Sunday. We went home a little early so I could get away from the crowds of people and get some rest. When we got there, I took off my hat and headband to show Shelly my stubbly head. She didn't seem too upset when she saw me and even suggested that I let her shave my head to remove the patches of stubble. I agreed to let her do this. I watched in the mirror and neither of us spoke as she slowly and gently shaved my head. When she finished she hugged me as the tears flowed softly once again.

Sunday was Shelly's birthday. She had gone back to her house on Saturday night, but we planned to meet at The Cheesecake Factory to really celebrate her 29th birthday. We got up early on Sunday so we could go to church (more crowds), but I really needed to go. I needed to worship and give praise and thanks for all of our prayers being answered and for the prayers of the people who were so caring and concerned for me. I decided to wear my wig. I tried to make it look as natural and as much like my style as possible, but the wig hair was a little longer than mine. I kept putting it on and taking it off until finally, I just put it on and gave it a good shake and made the "Fonzie" gesture to the mirror and we went out the door.

We arrived at church a little late because I had spent so much time on my no hair. My friend Jamie was a little late, too. As we both got out of our cars, she looked at me a little strange and then she said, "Oh, I like your hair". I didn't realize how upset I would be when confronted with this situation. As I looked at her, she could tell I was fighting back tears as I told her that it was a wig. All my hair had come out from the chemo treatment. She just hugged me and said she couldn't even tell it was a wig. How diplomatic and compassionate of her. It gave me a sense of calmness as we entered the sanctuary together. What a blessing to be in the Lord's house on the Lord's Day.

HAPPY BIRTHDAY SHELLY!

The Cheesecake Factory was one of Shelly's favorite places to eat. Of course, her birthday, May 5th, is also the Mexican Holiday, Cinco de Mayo. So there were always a lot of people celebrating on her birthday. We used to pretend that they were all celebrating her birthday. We had a great time at The Cheesecake Factory, but we were all so stuffed that we had no room for cheesecake. Shelly wasn't about to leave without the famous, and her favorite, Tiramisu Cheesecake. So, we ordered her some to go. Even after all the food we had at the weekend festivities, Richard and I ordered our favorite to take home, too! For me I ordered White Chocolate Macadamia Nut Cheesecake and for Richard, Chocolate Peanut Butter Cheesecake. It was a fun time together and a good memory to store for later.

TREATMENT #2

Monday morning we were all back to reality since we had to go to work. With my office in the basement, I had no excuse to stay home from work, even though I was feeling pretty exhausted from the weekend. I had a lot to do during the first two weeks of the month. There were lots of month-end reports to prepare and send out to whoever needed them. It was going to take all of my energy to focus on and do all of the tasks at hand. On top of that, my second chemo was in two days! I was just praying for physical strength to be able to accomplish all the things that needed to be done.

I worked all day Monday and Tuesday, taking short rest breaks to pace myself during the day. My treatment was scheduled at 12:45 PM on Wednesday, so I was able to work until about noon. I had been wearing the hats, headbands, scarves and turbans because I really didn't like the wig and Richard disliked it even more. But it would be hard to wear a hat and sit in the recliner for the treatment, so I decided to try the wig again. Shelly had asked for the afternoon off so she could be with us during this second treatment. The school was very good about letting her off whenever she needed it. My employer was very understanding about the time I had to be out of the office. I was told I could take whatever time was necessary and whenever necessary.

When we arrived at the oncologist's office, Shelly was already there. I registered at the desk and then waited for them to call my name. We all found a magazine to read while we waited. Once I was called back, the first thing they needed was a CBC to check and make sure that my red and white blood cell counts were back up. The nurse inserted a special needle that would remain in my arm during the entire treatment. The blood test would determine if I would be able to take the treatment or not. Fortunately, the blood counts were within range for me to be able to take the chemo.

After the blood test, I was sent to another waiting room (I called it the auxiliary waiting room) where Richard and Shelly were waiting for me. There we waited to see the doctor (more magazines). When my name was called, we all went into the exam room and the doctor did a routine check of my breast and asked what kind of problems I had been having. I told her that I had taken the medication for nausea and that, so far, I had suffered some nausea, but never to the point of throwing up. I told her that my hair had started coming out so we just shaved it all off and I asked, "Do you like my wig?" Of course, she said it was beautiful. I told her that my taste buds had disappeared for a little over two weeks, but they finally came back in time for my Dad's and Shelly's birthday celebrations. I told her about being in all of the crowds and she cautioned me to be careful in the future, because I didn't need to get any kind of an infection during the treatments. I told her that I would be more careful in the future. She once again checked my mouth for sores and asked if I had a sore throat. I was happy to report that I did not have either. She suggested that I buy a special mouthwash called Biotene to use to gargle and rinse out my mouth. This would help to prevent a sore throat and getting any sores in my mouth. Most people get these conditions during chemo treatments. So I had been very fortunate so far, even after being exposed to so many people.

After the exam, we were all ushered back to the chemotherapy room to begin the second treatment. I was still feeling very anxious about the procedure. The chemotherapy technician was preparing the concoction that I would be getting and in the meantime a nurse was preparing an IV drip with the pre-medications to prevent a reaction and nausea. When she came over to start the procedure she asked my name and what was my scheduled procedure for today. I told her that I would be having Adriamycin and Cytoxan chemotherapy today and it would be my second treatment of four. She was very careful to verify the pre-medications before continuing. As before, it took about thirty minutes for the pre-medications to go through the IV; then it was time for the chemotherapy. Once again the nurse asked my name and verified that I would be receiving the Adriamycin using the push method instead of the drip. She attached a tube to the butterfly needle, which had been left in my arm from the earlier CBC. Then she attached the large syringe filled with the red substance, Adriamycin. She sat there for over an hour and she slowly pushed the chemo into my arm. I could feel it going in because it was cooler than my body temperature. The nurse talked to me and to Richard and Shelly, who were sitting nearby. She would ask questions about things that were not at all related to the procedure, which helped to keep me from thinking about what I was going through. Once she finally finished with "Big Red" it was time for the Cytoxan. Once again they asked my name and verified the medication in the bag. Another tube was attached to the butterfly needle and the drip procedure was started.

Richard and Shelly took a break, and while they were gone I began to notice all of the other people in the chemotherapy room who were getting their treatment today as well. Some were ladies who looked to be about my age, some were much younger, some were older and a few were men, all receiving their treatments to battle their particular cancer. I began to talk with the ladies on either side of me. We shared our stories with each other and empathized with one another. Some had family members with them, but some did not. I felt sorry for the ones who didn't have anyone with them. I didn't think I could go through the treatment without someone from my family with me, but they seemed to manage just fine and I thought about how brave they were.

Once all of the Cytoxan had made its way into my body, the nurse changed the drip bag to another tube and began to push a saline solution through to clear my veins. This was the last step of the treatment. The nurse said that I should make an appointment for Friday so they could check my blood counts again. We stopped at the front desk and made the appointment for noon on Friday, so I could work up to my lunch hour and then go for the CBC.

By now it was about 5:00 PM and we knew that it was rush hour, so we decided to stop at the nearest restaurant to get something to eat before we went home. I did not really want anything to eat, but I thought I would try to eat something anyway. Shelly had dinner with us and then headed back home. By the time we finished with dinner, the traffic had subsided and we made it home without any problem. I was really tired when we got home and I was feeling nauseous, so I took the Zofran and just went straight to bed.

WIPED OUT!

I was able to work on Thursday, but I was still feeling drained of energy. The fatigue was a direct result of the chemo, which wiped out my red and white blood cells. This meant that I was probably not getting enough oxygen to my body. When I arrived for my CBC on Friday, I still wasn't feeling much better. Sure enough, the test revealed that my red blood cells and my white blood cells were way below normal. They gave me a Procrit shot to boost my red blood cells and also a Leukine shot to help boost my white blood cells. The nurse explained to me that the Leukine shot was the first of ten shots that would need to be taken daily. She also explained to me that my insurance would not pay for a nurse to give me the other nine shots, so I would need to do it myself! I was given a video to watch when I got home that would explain in detail how to give myself the shot. I was not a happy camper. I had never ever looked at the needle when I got a shot, but if I had to give it to myself, then I would have to look at it. The oncologist's office phoned in the prescriptions to my regular pharmacy, but the pharmacists did not have any on hand. They could order it that day and it would be there by the next day. The reason they did not keep it on hand was because it cost $300 per shot! That would mean it would cost $3,000 for 10 days of shots! WOW! Cancer is not cheap. Thank goodness my insurance would cover the medication even if it wouldn't cover the nurse's labor for giving the injection.

When I got home, I immediately watched the video to see what I would need to do. It seemed simple enough. Two good suggestions were to use ice on the injection site to numb the area and also, place a brand new needle on the syringe just before injecting the medication. This way you have a very sharp needle, not one that had already been used to penetrate the vile of medicine. I watched the video at least five times just to be sure I would know how to do this. I put it away and went downstairs to finish my work for the day.

We were able to get the nine vials (one for each day) of Leukine at the pharmacy the next day. Fortunately, I only had to pay the co-pay for prescriptions. I was more than a little anxious about giving myself the shot, so I played the video once again to be sure that I would know what I was doing. Finally, I said to myself, "Just do it." I went through all of the steps and once it was over I realized it wasn't so bad after all. One down and eight more to go!

I was not faring as well as I had with my first chemo. I was feeling tired, and I really didn't want anything to eat. I had to force myself to eat at every meal because I knew I needed to keep up my strength. I thought maybe it could be a build-up of the chemo in my system that was making me feel bad. I hoped and prayed that I would feel better tomorrow, because it would be Mother's Day.

HAPPY MOTHER'S DAY

Shelly had come to the house on Saturday to spend the night with us since it would be Mother's day on Sunday. Thankfully, by the time she got there my prayers were answered and I was feeling some better. She had bought me some new hats and headbands so I could have several different ones to wear during the months before my hair would grow back. They were so chic and stylish. I wouldn't mind wearing them at all.

My sister, Marilyn, and I had planned to take lunch to my Mother's house for Mother's Day. My Dad had surgery for removal of the end of one of his toes during the week before. So we wanted to do something to help them both. The surgery was a result of his diabetes. He had already had one toe removed on his left foot, so this was the second surgery on that foot. He was doing very well. Everyone seemed to enjoy the lunch and it was another great day of celebrating!

MAIL ORDER WIG

I was continuing to wear the expensive wig I had bought, but I was really not pleased at all with it. I decided I would go on the internet and see if there was anything else available. I found a website for a company called The Wig Company. I ordered a catalog so I could actually see the colors and styles they had available. When the catalog came, I picked a wig that I thought really looked like me and that was almost a perfect match to my hair color. To my surprise, the cost was less than fifty dollars even including the shipping. I placed the order and it arrived in about a week. I did not tell Richard or Shelly about it, so when I put it on for the first time, they asked what I had done to my wig because it looked so much better. When I told them it was a mail order wig that cost less than fifty dollars, they couldn't believe it. After that, I only wore this new wig, and I just put the expensive wig away.

BOOSTER SHOTS

I continued with my daily injections of the Leukine to help boost my white blood cells. I was to take the shots until Friday, May 17th, which was the 10th day after my chemo. I still felt tired and I just didn't feel like doing anything. I had no appetite at all and I just felt generally bad. I gave myself the last shot on the morning of the 10th day following my chemo. I was scheduled for another CBC that day and I was hoping that the results would be good. They were able to run the results of the test immediately, and the results showed that I was back to normal on all counts; but I wondered why I was still feeling so bad. I guessed that this is what it was going to be like.

I wasn't scheduled for another blood test until the following Thursday. The oncologist wanted to be sure that my counts were still good before it was time for my next chemo. By the time I returned to the office for this test, I was feeling so much better. It seemed that once I stopped taking the shots, I began to feel better and better each day. My test results were still good, so I was very thankful that I didn't have to have more Leukine shots before my next treatment.

LYNN REMEMBERED

Saturday, May 25th, was the anniversary of Lynn's death. It had been eighteen years since we had lost our beautiful daughter. I had finally gotten to the point where I could get through the day without crying. I knew that I would see Lynn again, in heaven. I was thinking that whatever happens with the cancer, it would be a win-win situation. If I survived, I would spend more time with Shelly and Richard and if I didn't, I would be spending eternity with Lynn. That thought gave me peace that day and I realized that I might hold that thought so that whenever I got discouraged I could call it to mind to lift my spirits. We always took live flowers to her grave and replaced the silk flowers in the marker vase with new ones as well. We would take items with us to clean the grave and the memorial bench that had been placed in the cemetery near her grave. It had been engraved with "In Loving Memory of Lynn Anderson—The Bottoms and Anderson Families". Richard's Mother had purchased the memorial shortly after Lynn died. Tending her grave was something that we could do for her and for ourselves. It was part of the grief process which had never really ended for us, and it probably never will.

TREATMENT #3

I was scheduled for my third chemotherapy treatment on the following Wednesday, May 29th. We followed the same routine as before, working Monday, Tuesday and until noon on Wednesday, and then we left to go to the oncology lab. On the way to the lab, Richard asked if I had changed clothes. I told him that I had not changed clothes but just added the jacket. He said he hadn't noticed what I had been wearing but thought something was different. I just looked at him and said, "I bet you wouldn't even notice if my hair fell out!" He looked at me and we both laughed out loud.

You would think that I would be getting use to this by now, but I was still having a lot of anxiety about the treatment. Once again, the nurse found a vein and inserted a butterfly needle which would be used later for the chemo. She filled a tube with enough blood for another CBC to be sure my counts were still OK before starting the third treatment. Everything was good to go and in about three hours we finished the treatment without any problems once again. Praise the Lord! The treatment time was shorter now that they knew I was not having any severe reactions to the drugs.

I reported back to the lab on Friday, May 31st to check my counts and sure enough, they were wiped out again. They gave me another Procrit shot and the Leukine shot. Another prescription was phoned to the pharmacy for the remainder of the Leukine. I had been using my thighs as the location for the shots, moving around in a circle on the right thigh for five shots and then switching to my left thigh for the remaining four shots. I was getting good at giving the shot, but I was still feeling bad just like before. I didn't want anything to eat because everything I ate tasted like cardboard. One day I asked Richard if he would go to the grocery store and get me some cottage cheese. Maybe it would taste normal to me because it always tasted like cardboard anyway; besides it was some protein and it would be good for me. I could live on that until my taste buds returned.

CHAPTER THREE

THE SUMMER MONTHS

MISTAKEN IDENTITY

On Wednesday, June 5th, I was back at the lab for my "10th day after chemo" blood test. My blood counts were improving. The Procrit and Leukine shots seemed to be working. I had just completed the last of this round of Leukine shots that day. My taste buds were back. I was thankful for every little victory, and I praised God for His care and for answered prayer.

On Friday, June 7th, I reported back to the lab for my usual CBC, and of course my counts were low. I was given another Procrit shot and started on another round of Leukine. I also had a follow-up appointment with the surgeon who had performed my biopsy and had diagnosed my condition as Inflammatory Breast Cancer. We went directly from the lab to her office. I brought her up to date on all that had happened. She performed a physical exam on my right breast and she agreed that the tumor was shrinking. This was very encouraging to me. Now I had confirmation from another doctor. She decided that she would order a ultrasound to check the progress of the reduction of the tumor.

I was moved to another room where the ultrasound would be performed. The technician was very kind and she had even warmed the gel that is used on the ultrasound instrument that is placed against the skin (thank goodness!). She spent a long time trying to pick up some kind of an image of the tumor. Finally after about thirty minutes she completed the procedure. I got dressed and was ushered back into the surgeon's office. She already had the results from the technician. She told me that she was not able to determine how much the tumor had diminished because the technician could not get anything definitive to show up on the ultrasound. Apparently this type of tumor is very illusive. This type of tumor grows in sheets instead of a lump.

My mind immediately flashed back to the ultrasound, which had been done at the radiologist's office in the very beginning. The technician there had also tried for forty-five minutes to get an image of the tumor but was unsuccessful. Then I remembered that the radiologist had detected the tumor with a mammogram. I suggested to the surgeon that maybe we should try a mammogram because that is how it was originally detected. The surgeon just looked at me and said that she had seen that mammogram. She said there was no way anyone could tell from that mammogram that I had a tumor of any kind, much less a malignant tumor. She told me that the radiologist had been mistaken. I could not believe what she was saying! I told her that I had seen it on the screen and the radiologist had told me that it was at the five o'clock position! She said the only thing that showed up at that position was some calcification, which was nothing to worry about. My tumor was between ten and two o'clock. I said, "But your biopsy confirmed that I have a malignant tumor!" She just shrugged her shoulders and said, "I know, but it did not show up on the mammogram!"

If that radiologist had been mistaken, I sure was thankful that he was. He got my attention and by doing so I was able to get to a surgeon as soon as I possibly could. I was in shock and awe and total amazement! I suddenly realized that God had a hand in my diagnosis! I had been blessed in an unusual way, a miraculous way and all of a sudden I was so humbled by everything that had taken place! All things ARE possible with God as our Creator!

CBC, CBC, CBC!

During all of this time of blood tests, chemotherapy treatments, shots, ultrasound, wigs, hats and headbands, I was still trying to get my work done in my office. With all of the doctor appointments, I found myself working a lot at night in order to stay caught up. I still was not feeling good at all. I did feel nauseous sometimes, but I never got to the point of actually throwing up (for me, that's right before dying). The bad feeling was more like I had a virus or the flu. I guess that's the way chemo affects most people. But usually by the eleventh or twelfth day after the treatment, I would begin to feel better. My taste buds would start functioning again and for a few days, I really enjoyed eating and tasting food again. My energy level was still low, and I had to pace myself in order to work through a whole day. My sister, Ann, would come over and help me get caught up when I would get off schedule. She was a big help to me. I couldn't have done it without her.

On Wednesday, June 12th, it was time for another CBC to see how those cute little blood cells were coming along. To my dismay, my red cells and white cells had dropped in only a week's time and I hadn't even had any chemo since the last blood test. This couldn't be good. The oncologist prescribed a very strong antibiotic because my counts were so low. She also wanted me to have another Procrit shot and to resume the Leukine shots at home. These steps would hopefully bring my counts back up before June 19th when it would be time for my fourth and final A/C treatment.

Once I started back with the Leukine shots, I started feeling bad again. I suddenly realized that maybe the Leukine was what was making me feel this way. I continued to give myself the shots and decided I would mention it to my oncologist on the next visit. I also began having a very high fever. I was still taking the antibiotic so that was all that could be done except take a fever reducer like Tylenol.

June 16th was Father's Day, so we celebrated with Richard and then went to my Mom and Dad's house to celebrate with them. We brought the family up to date on my blood cell count situation and we just asked everyone to keep praying for us.

On Monday, June 17th, I reported once again to the lab for another CBC. The counts were improving but still not enough to have chemo on Wednesday, so I was instructed to continue with the Leukine shots. I decided not to mention the fact that I thought the Leukine was making me feel bad.

The next day, I was scheduled to have my Annual Pap Test and Physical Exam. This was the appointment that I had made way back in April when I first tried to see my gynecologist for the problem I was having with my right breast. Thank goodness I didn't wait until later to get something done. I would be seeing this doctor for the very first time. He had been notified of the diagnosis and when I saw him I brought him up to date as much as I could without taking too much time. The usual tests were performed and I was promised that I would be notified of the results within seven to ten days.

The very next day I was scheduled to have my fourth chemotherapy treatment. It would be my final A/C treatment. When I arrived at the lab the first thing they did, as usual, was to take a CBC. As we waited for the results we were all praying that I would be able to take the treatment today. I really wanted to get this series over with and go on to the next round of four more treatments. When the results came back, the white cell counts were still too low and it was decided that the treatment would have to be cancelled. Richard and I both were so disappointed. I never thought I would feel that way about a chemotherapy treatment, but I did. I was advised to continue taking my antibiotic and the Leukine shots until Monday and then come back for another CBC.

That night as I was getting ready for bed, I noticed that I had developed a reddish rash all over my legs and my arms. This was very upsetting to me. I had been given a number that I could call anytime during the day or night if I needed to ask questions or if I was having a problem. I decided to call this "nurse line" and report the situation. When I called, the nurse asked what kind of medications I was taking and I told her that I was taking Leukine and an antibiotic called Levequin. She said more than likely I was having a reaction to the antibiotic. She advised me to stop taking it and to take some Benadryl to treat the symptoms of the reaction. She advised me to call my oncologist in the morning.

By morning my rash had turned into little white blisters all over my legs and arms and I even had some on my torso. I called the doctors office and left word that I thought I was having a reaction to the antibiotics and that, on the advice of the person on the "nurse line," I had stopped taking them for now. My oncologist called back and said that she would prescribe another antibiotic and that I should take Benadryl to treat the symptoms of the reactions. I told her I was already taking the Benadryl. I had an appointment for another CBC on Monday. This was Thursday.

By Saturday, all of my little white blisters had begun to pop and my skin was peeling off my legs and arms. I looked like I had been doused in a vat of flour. I applied moisturizer to my skin to make it feel a little better and it did help some. I couldn't help feeling a little sorry for myself. What else could happen? For the first time I found myself crying from the inside out. When Richard came to see what was wrong I just told him that I was feeling sorry for myself. He asked me not to cry and I told him that this was my pity-party and I could cry if I wanted to! I deserved to have a good cry! If he couldn't take it he could just go somewhere else. He just went downstairs to his office and waited it out. Pretty soon all my tears were cried out, and I was OK after that.

I reported to the lab on Monday for another CBC to see how my counts were coming along. Fortunately they were improving and it was very likely that I could resume my treatments on Wednesday. The first layer of my skin had just about all peeled off by now and I was looking a lot better. My oncologist told me not to let anyone give me Levequin again since I had had this type of reaction.

On Wednesday, June 26th, I returned to the lab and, as usual, another CBC was taken. The results were good enough for me to go ahead with the treatment.

I was actually glad about this. So once again we went through the three-hour routine. I was scheduled for another CBC on Friday, so we returned to the lab on Friday and to no one's surprise, my red and white cells were wiped out. I was given another Procrit shot and I was advised to continue with the daily Leukine shots for the next ten days. I told my oncologist that I thought the Leukine shots were making me feel bad. She said that it was probably just the chemotherapy. I explained to her that when I had to start taking the Leukine again on the last visit, that I had started to feel bad and I didn't even have the chemo. She said that sometimes people cannot tolerate the Leukine and when that happens, she is then able to prescribe a new drug called Neulasta. With this drug you only have to take one shot, which could be administered by the nurse instead of the ten self-injected shots for ten days, but the one shot was very expensive. I asked her, "How much could it be, the ten Leukine shots were $3,000.00?" She said the one shot would cost $4,900.00! The insurance company would not pay for it unless it was proven that the patient could not tolerate the Leukine, which was the drug of choice (the insurance company's choice, that is). Like I said, cancer is not cheap. I was given the Neulasta shot that day. I was to return the following Friday for another CBC to check the results.

NEW SIDE EFFECTS

By late Saturday afternoon, I had begun to have a severe backache. I tried to lay flat on the floor with my feet up on the sofa to try to get some relief. It hurt constantly. Then I began to hurt in my shoulders, too. I thought that I must have strained a muscle or maybe a disc had slipped out of place or maybe I was getting the flu. That's what it felt like. I was beginning to ache all over just like when you have the flu, but ten times worse. I took some Tylenol, but it didn't seem to help much. I told Richard that I thought I might need to go to the Chiropractor for an adjustment, to see if that wouldn't help the pain. It was Saturday, so I would have to wait until Monday before I could get to the Chiropractor.

The pain continued unrelentingly, so I continued to take Tylenol, which did help a little. I finally decided to call the "nurse line" again and report this problem. When I explained to the nurse what was happening, she asked what medications I was taking and I told her about the Zofran, Procrit, Neulasta and now Tylenol for the bone pain. She said that the pain was caused by the Neulasta injection. This medication stimulates the bone marrow to produce more white blood cells and it usually causes the bones to ache like you have the flu, but ten times worse. It usually affects the larger bones like the pelvis and the shoulderblades. She said that these side effects should have been explained to me when the medication was prescribed. I didn't remember anyone telling me this, but I was kind of relieved when she told me that it was the medication. I was beginning to think that the cancer might have already spread to my bones. She suggested that I continue to take Tylenol for the time being, and she would have the doctor phone the pharmacy for a prescription for some pain medication. She said that I should be able to pick it up the next day, which was Sunday, July1st.

HAPPY FOURTH OF JULY!

I was so glad to be finished with the first round of the Adriamycin and Cytoxan treatments. The weather was predicted to be beautiful for the annual 4th of July and the traditional Thomas Memorial Antique Steam Powered Tractor Parade in our local town of Cumming, GA. It was a huge event for the whole county. Everyone came from miles around to see the steam engines that powered the huge tractors of yesteryear. It was the same type of engines that were used on locomotives to move them across the country. Farmers used them to power the tractors, which planted, plowed and harvested their crops. Of course this was before the gasoline engines came along. I was really looking forward to going this year. After all, I hadn't missed a parade since Lynn was a baby. It was a carnival atmosphere with all kinds of food and fun. Since the new fairgrounds had been opened, everyone would go there after the parade to participate in the festivities. You could get funnel cakes and corn dogs and cotton candy. The smell of barbequed chicken and pork filled the air. It was always an exciting event.

SECOND ROUND COMING UP

With each chemotherapy treatment, my blood cell counts seemed to be lower and lower. My body was really taking a hit from the treatments. It would take a while for the Neulasta shot to take effect and build up the white blood cells. I was still having a lot of bone pain from the shot, so we were just praying that the Neulasta was working. The prescription for the pain medication had really helped. When we woke up on Thursday, July 4th, I was really feeling tired. I really wanted to go to the parade; but if my counts were low then I shouldn't be in a crowd of people, and there was always a big crowd at the parade. We decided that I needed to stay home and just rest and try to get my strength back. It was disappointing, but I knew it was the best thing for me to do. I was scheduled for another CBC on the next day, so it wouldn't be long until we would find out if the Neulasta was working.

We showed up at the lab early in the morning on the 5th as scheduled, and once again it took a needle-stick or two to find a vein. I noticed that most people that were taking chemotherapy had what was called a "port". This device had to be implanted surgically under outpatient conditions. It looked like a nickel just under the skin. Once the port was implanted, it was not necessary to get a needle stick in the skin to find a vein. The port was used each time a blood test was needed or a treatment was administered. I was feeling kind of left out because I didn't have one, so I decided on my next visit to my oncologist, I would ask her why I didn't have one.

We waited in the auxiliary waiting room for the lab technician to run the test results for the CBC. When the nurse came out to discuss the results, I could tell by the look on her face that it was not good. The normal range for the white blood cells should be 4.8-10.8. Mine was only 0.6. On top of that problem, the normal range for the new baby white blood cells called neutrophyls was 2.00-8.00. My count was 0.11! That meant that my white cells were very low, and even the new baby white cells were not being produced yet.! My immune system was just about non-existent right then. Of course I was given another antibiotic which I was to begin taking immediately, and I was again advised to stay away from crowds and especially from small children. I was to come back in 5 days, which would be Wednesday, July 10th, to have another CBC. I could not take another Neulasta shot until after my next chemo treatment. I don't know if that was because of the insurance company's policies or because of the possibility of incompatible drug specifications. We would have to wait until the following Wednesday to see if my immune system would be restored.

On Wednesday, July 10th, off we went to the lab once more. I tried to schedule these blood tests during my lunch hour, so I could work as much as possible. My white cells had jumped from 0.6 to 3.7. That was good but still below the normal range. The good news was that the neutrophyls had jumped from 0.11 to 58.8!! So, in a few days these would mature into adult white blood cells. I was recovering and I was praising the Lord!

On Friday, July 12th, I had been scheduled to have a CT Scan of my chest and abdomen at 7:30 AM. Hopefully this would give us some idea of the progress that was being made on the tumor after completing the first four A/C chemotherapy treatments. We would also be taking a look at the spots that had shown up on my liver during the first CT Scan in April. The results were to be ready by the following Tuesday. The oncologist called on Tuesday, July 16th and gave us some good news. The spots on my liver had not changed and there was no evidence that the cancer had spread. Praise the Lord and Glory Hallelujah!! However, the scan still was not able to get a definitive image of the tumor. I was to report the next day for my fifth chemotherapy treatment, which would be the first of four treatments of the drug called Taxotere. My oncologist advised me to begin taking my pre-medication dose of benadryl that night to help prevent any allergic reaction to the new chemo.

On Wednesday, July 17th, I reported to the lab and went through the same routine of CBC and pre-medications to prevent nausea and allergic reaction. Then the Taxotere was started, which only took about 2 hours. I had a chance to ask the oncologist if I could get a port so I wouldn't have to be stuck so many times. I told her that I had noticed that most everyone had one and that I was feeling left out. She said that as long as I could tolerate the sticks and they were able to get a vein, she would not recommend that a port be implanted. The process would be an outpatient surgery that would be performed at the hospital, and there were a lot of problems that could go along with a port. A patient could develop an infection at the port site, or they could develop a blood clot that could cause a number of other serious complications. The doctor said she would rather that I not have a port at that time. Because I knew that I should keep myself hydrated as much as possible before the procedure, I was not having too much difficulty with the nurse finding a vein. I had started drinking lots of water two days before a blood test or chemo treatment was scheduled. After talking it over with my physician, I was satisfied not to have the procedure and to just continue as we were doing until (if and when) it became necessary for me to have a port.

I finished the treatment by 2:00 PM that day. I had been informed of a support group that met every Wednesday from 2:00-3:00 PM. The group was led by my friend who had gotten the appointment for me to obtain a second opinion regarding the best regime of treatments, which led me to secure the physician who ultimately became my oncologist. Shelly was with me that day, and when I asked her if she could go with me, she agreed. When we arrived at the meeting, it was already in progress. Each person was allowed to give their name and to tell the type of cancer for which they were being treated, and to share problems they were having or anything else they wanted to talk about. When it was my turn, I shared with the group the fact that I was ready for the chemo treatments to be finished. When Shelly's turn came, she said that she didn't mean to sound selfish, but that she didn't want the chemo treatments to be over for me, because then nothing would be fighting the cancer. This was the first time the group had heard this perspective from a family member. We all learned a lot that day about other people and all of the problems and disappointments that they had been facing. Somehow, it made my problems not seem so overwhelming. I don't mean to say that it was comforting that other people were suffering, but it was comforting to know that I was not alone on the journey. There was laughter and there were tears as everyone shared their stories. My friend was very helpful and encouraging to each and every one that was there. I decided that I would try to attend the support group meeting whenever I was able to do so.

MOUNTAIN GET-A-WAY

I usually had to go back to the lab on Friday, following each of my chemo treatments on Wednesday, for a Neulasta shot and a Procrit shot; but we had been invited to stay at a mountain home that belonged to one of the owners of the company for which I was working. He was so generous and kind to offer it to us. So I was allowed to come back after 2:00 PM on Thursday (you have to wait at least twenty four hours after chemo before you can take the Neulasta shot) in order to get a Procrit shot and a Neulasta shot. We were to leave early on Friday morning to meet the Vice President and his lovely wife at their beautiful home in Cashiers, North Carolina. I was actually excited about the trip. I am the mountain person in our family. Richard and Shelly always like to go to the beach.

If anyone has ever been driving in the mountains, you know how winding the roads can be. The Taxotere was not supposed to have the severe side effects that you have with the A/C treatments. I had taken my nausea medications before we left, but I was beginning to feel a little queasy on the way there. Richard said that it might just be the winding roads. Even a normal person could get carsick on the roads leading to Cashiers. Fortunately, we arrived about an hour before we were to have lunch, so by the time we were being seated at a restaurant just outside of Cashiers, I was feeling much better. We had a great time during lunch and also back at the house afterwards. Our host and hostess stayed until almost evening, and then left us there to spend Friday night and Saturday night on our own. It was so quiet and peaceful there. They had left plenty of food in the refrigerator for us, and we helped ourselves to some steaks on the grill for dinner. I made a nice salad and cooked baked potatoes in the microwave. The sun was setting just as we were finishing dinner. We watched some TV and then went to bed. The bedrooms were upstairs and our hostess had decorated them and named them in honor of President Thomas Jefferson and President George Washington. We decided to sleep in the Thomas Jefferson room. We got up and had breakfast the next morning and then went for a drive in the mountains. We saw lakes and streams and waterfalls and just really enjoyed the day. While we were driving back to the house, I began to have the bone pain from the Neulasta shot once again. I had not thought to bring my pain medication, but I did have some Tylenol with me and that helped some. When we got back to the mountain home it was late in the evening and we just got ready for bed. The night air was cool so we opened the windows, and we could hear all the sounds of the mountains, and you could actually see the stars because there were no city lights or street lights to block the view. We got up early on Sunday and started the winding road trip back home. It really had been great to get away to the peace and quietness of the beautiful mountains for a few days.

SECOND THOUGHTS

On the way home from the mountains, I somehow started thinking about the fact that I could be having surgery now instead of waiting for another three months to have this cancer or what was left of it taken out. The goal was to shrink it to an operable size and then remove it if there was anything left of it by the time I was to have the surgery. All of a sudden I just wanted the treatments to be over, and the sooner the better. The longer the cancer was there the more chances it would have to spread. At the time we made the decision, we all agreed that this would be the best course of treatment. Now, I was having second thoughts and I was becoming very agitated about the situation. I was just hoping and praying that we had not made a mistake by choosing this option. I finally just turned it over to the Lord and put my trust in Him for the days ahead.

BACK TO ROUTINE

When we got home on Sunday afternoon, I had work waiting for me, and so did Richard. We were both tired from the trip back, so we just put everything away and took advantage of the last part of this day of rest. We went to bed early because we would need to be up early to tackle the list of things that we needed to get done. You know the old saying "Early to bed, early to rise, makes a man *healthy*, wealthy and wise".

I did not have to report for a CBC until Friday, July 26th, so we spent the week trying to get caught up at work and at home. My lab appointment wasn't until 12:00 noon on Friday, so I was able to work right up to the time I had to leave. I always expected my blood cell counts would be good every time I went for a CBC, but of course they never were. I guess you could call me the proverbial optimist. This time however, the Neulasta had really been doing its job. In only one month my white cell count had gone from 3.69 to 29.4! That meant no antibiotics for me this time! Finally, I could say that all of the bone pain from the Neulasta was really worth it. My red blood cells were still a little below normal, so I was given a Procrit shot to boost them before my next treatment, which would be on Wednesday, August 7th. Until then I would be waiting for my taste buds to start functioning again; and we planned that when they did, we would go out to have a nice dinner and celebrate these little victories.

During the month of August I would have my sixth and seventh Taxotere treatments and the usual CBC's followed by Neulasta and Procrit shots. The only unexpected event was a problem with my right eye. I could see what looked like a fly flittering in front of me all the time. I was afraid that the chemo might be affecting my eyesight, so I made an appointment for an eye examination on Tuesday, August 20th, at 4:45PM. I explained to the doctor that I had been having chemo and about the fly in front of my face all the time. He did a thorough exam and afterwards explained the condition. Apparently this is a common malady whether you are taking chemo or not. I had what is called a *floater* in my eye. It was caused by a small piece of the tissue in the eye flaking off due to dryness, which could have been a result of the chemo because it does have a drying affect on your skin. It also could have been due to the dreaded condition of "aging". Whatever the cause, there was really nothing that could be done about it now. Sometimes these things dissolve on their own and disappear. If not, I would eventually become so use to the speck being there that I wouldn't even notice it.

The time was drawing nearer and nearer for my last chemo treatment. Only one more to go! I was looking forward to having the treatments behind me and then going on to the next step. I was still trusting God for strength and peace and healing and comfort not only for me but for Richard and Shelly, too.

YOU LOOK SO GOOD!

From the time I began taking chemo, almost everyone with whom I came in contact would ask me how I was doing. I would describe to each person the most current activity. Inevitably every person would tell me that I really looked good after all I had been going through. At first I was really glad to hear this. I was almost proud of the fact that I was able to maintain my composure and even with a wig people were very complimentary. But after awhile, I began to feel that no one really thought that I was having any difficulty whatsoever because I always "looked so good". Then one day we went to the funeral of a friend of ours who had passed away. We stayed quite awhile, and during that time I noticed that almost everyone, including me, who came to pay respects to the family and to the person who had passed away would say "He really looks good." After that, my attitude really went downhill. Every time someone said that I really looked good, all I could think was that those were the words people say when you are lying in state at your funeral. I told Richard that if I heard one more person say that to me, I thought I would just scream.

In between all of the treatments and tests, I was still working. We had a luncheon planned at my company's club, which we had frequented quite a bit over the years. During that time we had become familiar with one of the servers who had been there a long time, so we always asked for him to be our server. With everything that had been going on, it had been quite a while since we had a chance to dine at the club. As a matter of fact, this would be the first time since my diagnosis. When our server came by to take my order, he looked at me a little strangely, and he said "You look different, have you been sick or something?" I was so surprised that I almost didn't know what to say. He was from another country and really did not know that what he said would upset me. He was just telling the truth. Finally, I did manage to tell him that, as a matter of fact, I had been sick, that I had breast cancer and I was taking chemotherapy treatments. He expressed his concern and hoped that I would recover. I thanked him and we continued with the luncheon. When I got home, I just wanted to cry. I told Richard that someone had finally told me the truth about the way I looked and it had really upset me and that I would never again complain about anyone saying "You look so good". I had a whole new attitude and a whole new outlook.

CHAPTER FOUR

THE MONTH OF SEPTEMBER

CONSULTATION FOR SURGERY

On Wednesday, September 4th, I was scheduled for a consultation with my dear surgeon who had performed my first biopsy. As we were driving to her office I couldn't help thinking back to the day she called me and gave me the diagnosis, and told me the tumor was inoperable, and had referred me to an oncologist. It had been five months since I had heard the words "malignant tumor" applied to me. I had completed seven chemo treatments since April 19th (one every three weeks, except for the one that was delayed for one week).

When I finally got in to see my surgeon, she was almost as excited as I was that so much progress had been made in the reduction of the tumor, and that it was now possible to undergo surgery to remove what was left of it, if any! She said that I would be having a Modified Radical Mastectomy of the right breast and removal of the auxillary lymph nodes on Thursday, October 17th at Northside Hospital Women's Center at 1:00PM. My last chemo was scheduled for September 18th, and this would give me four weeks for my system to recover in order for me to withstand the surgery. It would be an overnight hospital stay and would be considered as outpatient surgery! She informed me that I would not be eligible for reconstructive surgery for at least six to twelve months due to the nature of this tumor, which is considered highly recurrent. However, she suggested that I schedule a consultation with a plastic surgeon before the surgery because they would want to make pictures and x-rays for future reference, that is, if and when I did decide to have reconstructive surgery. I ask her if she could recommend someone, and she gave me the name and number of the head of plastic surgery at Northside Hospital in Atlanta. I would need to call and schedule an appointment before October 17th.

I had some questions about the surgery, and one of them was about the bandages after the surgery. I don't know why I was so concerned about that, but I was. She said that I would have a clear, cellophane like strip over the incision. This would enable me to take a shower 48 hours after the surgery. I could not imagine that all I would have was a piece of clear tape over the incision after removing all of that tissue. I was thinking that I would have this big bulky gauze like bandage with something wrapped all the way around me to hold the bandages in place. How could they just put a Band-Aid on it? She did say that I would have a drain-tube coming out of the incision to allow the fluid that would accumulate to drain and prevent swelling and pain.

She indicated that I would have radiation treatments five days a week for seven weeks after the surgery. She said the prognosis for success of the surgery was good! That was really great to hear after all I had been through. She wanted to know if I was still working, and I told her "every day". She wanted to know how I had managed to handle this as well as I had. I told her that I had a lot of people praying for me and those prayers were being answered everyday, and that it was my Lord and Savior and Comforter who had sustained me and my family thus far. His promises are true. I was very much encouraged by her words that day. I praised God for the successes that we had and for the ones yet to come. When we got home from the surgeon's office, I called the plastic surgeon's office and was able to schedule an appointment for a consultation on October 4th.

I reported to the lab as scheduled on Friday, September 6th for yet another CBC. My white blood cells were amazingly high and even the red blood cells were almost up to the normal range. It was so great to have a good report and to not have to take more shots and medications just to be able to take one more treatment.

LYNN'S 35TH BIRTHDAY REMEMBERED

On Saturday, September 14th, we went to the florist to purchase fresh cut flowers to place on Lynn's grave. She would have been thirty-five years old. We also purchased new silk flowers to replace the ones that were in the vase of the grave marker. We usually replaced them about four times a year because it doesn't take long for the elements to fade the beautiful colors of the silk flower arrangements. We also cleaned the marker and the memorial bench that Richard's parents had placed in the cemetery near Lynn's grave. It gave us something to do for her, even though she was gone.

FINALLY, THE LAST TREATMENT!

On Wednesday, September 18th, I gladly entered the lab for my eighth and final chemotherapy treatment! This would be the last I would see of that needle (I still did not have a port). We had the usual CBC before chemo and my counts were very good, so on with the show! All was just routine for this last treatment and I was very thankful for that. When I finished the treatment the whole staff presented me with a Certificate of Achievement Special Merit Award. Everyone had signed it with good wishes and encouragement. I was so touched by it all that I began to cry. Everyone had been so good to me, and now I would be moving on to the next step. I felt like I would never see them again, but then I remembered I would have to have a CBC on Friday, and then I was OK.

I did return to the lab on Friday for my CBC, which showed that my white cell counts were wiped out as usual. So, I had another Neulasta shot to help boost the white cells. The red blood cells were better than usual but still below the normal range. I needed another Procrit shot, too, especially since I would be having surgery in four weeks. They wanted me to be in the best physical condition possible.

This same day, Friday, September 20th, was also Richard's birthday. He loves to go to the Japanese steak houses where they cook the food in front of you, so Shelly met us at our favorite one for dinner that night for the big celebration! We took some pictures that night at dinner. When we got home, I realized I only had a few frames left on the roll of film. Richard wanted to get a picture of both of us together with our bald heads showing. So, to make him happy I took off my wig, we stood in front of the bathroom mirror, we put our heads together then tilted them so that the tops of our heads were facing the camera. I held the camera and took the picture. I finished the roll and took it to one of those one-hour photo shops to have the film developed. When I got them back we hurriedly looked through them to find that particular picture. When we saw it, it looked like a baby's bottom! Apparently, I held the camera so close that it only picked up the very tops of our heads! It was so funny that we laughed until we hurt. We couldn't wait to show Shelly the picture.

September is always a very full month for us. We also celebrated our thirty-seventh wedding anniversary on the 25th of the month. Richard surprised me by taking me to the jewelry counter at Macy's. He had already picked out a diamond ring with three beautiful diamonds that represented the past, the present and the future. All that was needed was for me to have my finger measured so it could be sized. Not only was the ring beautiful, but so was the thought behind it! It was a celebration not only of our anniversary, but of also getting through the treatments. Now we were looking to the surgery that would hopefully be the cure, so that we could have a future together.

On Friday, September 27th, at 12:00 noon, I reported to the lab once more. This would be the last time I would have a CBC before surgery. My counts were good and I was "good to go!" I was scheduled for my first one-month check up on October 24th. This would be one week after the surgery. Because of the aggressiveness of this cancer, it would be necessary for me to come back once a month for one year for a follow-up appointment with the oncologist.

CHAPTER FIVE

THE MONTH OF OCTOBER

UNDER THE KNIFE

After completing my last treatment and taking my last booster shots, I was not scheduled for any appointments until October 3rd. On that day I was instructed to call Northside Hospital and complete a telephone assessment for surgery. The lady that I spoke with that day was so very nice. She asked all of the usual questions about name, address, medications, allergies and if I had had any prior surgeries. It only took about fifteen minutes and we were finished.

After I hung up the phone, I realized that I had never ever been "under the knife" before in my whole life. I had been with Richard when he had surgery for a cyst on the end of his spine and with Shelly when she had her tonsils and adenoids taken out, but I had never had anything like that. As a matter of fact, I had hardly ever been sick in my whole life other than the usual childhood diseases. The only one I could remember was the mumps. I am one of seven children. When my youngest brother, Henry, had gotten the mumps at school, the following week five of us came down with them. My sister, Ann, slept between me and Marilyn and she never did "catch" them from us. I only had swelling on one side but everyone else had both sides of their jaw swollen and very sore. When we all recovered and were planning on going back to school the next day, I woke up with the other side swollen, so I had to stay out of school another week.

I really liked going to school. I guess it was because it was a lot more fun than staying at home and helping with the endless chores that needed to be done for a family of nine. I do not know how my Mother handled it. She had seven children and the oldest was almost ten years old when the youngest was born. We lived on a farm and we raised hogs and cows and chickens and vegetables and kids. We always had fresh vegetables to eat and fresh milk from cows. We made butter from the cream that would rise to the top of the milk. I guess we always drank fat free milk and didn't realize it. Oh well, so much for childhood memories.

I guess I never really quite learned how to be sick. I worked almost every day while taking the chemotherapy treatments. Now with the surgery approaching, I knew that I would have to be out of work for a few days to recover. Surgery was scheduled to be on a Thursday, so I was hoping that I would be able to go downstairs to my office by the following Monday, that is if everything went OK. We were getting ready for a computer software conversion at work, and I did not want to be away from my job for very long.

LAST MINUTE CHECKLIST

There were three more things that I had to do before my surgery. First was the consultation with the plastic surgeon, which was scheduled for October 4th, second was my usual dental check up on the 14th, and the last thing was a class for breast cancer surgery patients, which was scheduled for the evening of the 14th at Northside Hospital where I would be having my surgery on Thursday the 17th.

On Friday, October 4th, Richard and I went to the plastic surgeon's office to which my surgeon had referred me. When we arrived, I was asked to fill out all of the usual new patient intake information, and then we were ushered back to the plastic surgeon's office. She talked with us about reconstruction procedures so that I could make an informed decision about it at a later time. She wanted to get some x-rays and some pictures of my breasts from several different angles so that she would have something to work from if I did want to have reconstruction at some point. I was given a release form, which I could choose to sign or not to sign, that would allow them to use these photographs to help show other women what could be done in reconstruction. At first, I didn't want to sign it. I didn't want pictures of my breast shown to anyone else, but then I realized that they would not be showing my face and that it would be helping other women to make a decision about whether or not to have reconstruction. I remember seeing the photos of the breasts of women who had Inflammatory Breast Cancer and the sacrifice that they had made to help inform people about this very rare and deadly cancer. So I decided that I would sign the release form in the hopes that it would be helpful to other women who were dealing with breast cancer. We made the pictures and the x-rays and had a final discussion with the plastic surgeon. She said that whenever I was ready, just call and make an appointment to come back to see her. As we left her office that day she wished me the best of success and good health.

On Monday, October 14th, I went for my six month dental check up. Sometimes chemotherapy can cause teeth and gum problems; but, thank goodness, they did not see any problems. I had the usual cleaning and exam and the hygienist wanted to take x-rays of my teeth. I asked her if we could wait until my next appointment, because I was going to be having a lot of radiation after my surgery. The dentist agreed to forego the x-rays this time and scheduled them for my next visit, which would be in six months.

On the evening of that same day, I drove to Northside Hospital for the class that would inform me about the procedures awaiting me on Thursday. There were a lot of other breast cancer patients there. The leader of the class walked us through all the procedures that would take place on the day of the surgery, starting with registration and ending with being assigned a room where we could stay until checkout time, which would be within 23 hours from the time we were registered, presuming everything went according to plans. All of the women in the class were preparing to have surgery. Some would have a lumpectomy, some a mastectomy and one lady was going to have a double mastectomy even though she only had cancer in one breast. Apparently she had a gene that is inherited (BRCA) that is linked to breast cancer, and by having the other breast removed now, she would be able to avoid the possibility of another bout with breast cancer in the future. I had a lot of questions and listened to everyone else's questions. We all learned a lot about what was going to happen through every step of our surgery. It was comforting and it relieved a lot of anxiety for all of us. In just the short time that we were all together, we became "bosom buddies" before we left for home.

I had continued to work everyday. My strength was returning and I was feeling better and better with each passing day. I was just counting down the days until surgery. I couldn't wait to get it over with.

SURGERY, FINALLY!

When the day finally arrived to have surgery, I got up early and tried to get some work done. I wasn't supposed to eat anything, so I tried to stay busy to take my mind off food. Now that I finally had my taste buds back, all I wanted to do was eat, and that day I wasn't allowed to. I had to report to the admissions office at the hospital at 1:00 PM for registration. When Richard, Shelly and I got there, a lot of my family were already there, waiting for us. My Mother, two sisters and two brothers were able to come to the hospital, and the new pastor from our church had come as well. A very good friend of ours, Dorris, who had arranged my very first date with Richard so many years ago, was also there. They came to wish me well, and to say prayers for me and my family during my surgery. I was glad, not only for my sake, but for Richard's and Shelly's sake as well. They would have someone with them while I was in surgery.

I had been preparing myself for this day through prayer, and with the prayers of others. I was just trusting the Lord to be with me and to guide the surgeon's hands. I knew that I would not be having reconstructive surgery, and I was trying not to think about how my body would be after the surgery. I was trying to focus on being free of this disease that had consumed my every waking moment since April 5th. I was not afraid, but I was a bit nervous. I know that Richard and Shelly were having a lot of anxiety about me going into surgery; yet with the Lord's help I was able to be calm and peaceful and by doing so, hopefully, I was able to calm their fears. I just turned my eyes upon Jesus and prayed that He would help me through this, and that everything would be OK when it was over.

The anesthesiologist came in to go over his part of the procedure with me. The surgery was scheduled to last about two hours; and then there would be some time in recovery, based upon when I came out of the anesthesia. Richard and Shelly were allowed to stay with me until I was given some medication that would relax me and make me sleepy. I was still awake when they rolled my gurney into the operating room. I remember that it was very cold and that I had to be lifted onto the operating table. I don't remember seeing my surgeon before I went completely under the anesthesia. I guess she was scrubbing for the surgery.

DID THEY GET IT ALL?

The surgery was scheduled to last about two hours; and then, of course, I would have some time in recovery. Richard and Shelly were instructed to wait in a special waiting-room nearby. They were to be updated at certain intervals of the surgery, either by phone or by someone in person. This would let them know how the surgery was progressing and how I was doing. Almost two hours went by, and they had not received any updates. Shelly would occasionally go out into the community waiting room, where everyone else was waiting, and let them know that they had not heard anything. They all were getting very anxious and there was a lot of pacing back and forth. Finally a nurse did come and update them. Apparently I had been bumped from my scheduled time and they were just now beginning the surgery, so it would be about two hours from then before I would be out of surgery. They did receive regular updates during the next two hours, which assured them that everything was going well. Then it was two-and-one-half hours, and then three, and no one was updating them. That's when the pacing really started. Finally the surgeon came and met with Richard and Shelly. My Mother had also been allowed to stay in the room while the surgeon talked with them. The news was not what they had hoped for. The surgeon said that she was not able to get clear margins in the skin on the lower side of the incision. In other words, they did not get it all! I think Richard and Shelly went into shock when she told them. My Mother could not hear very well, so Shelly had to explain it to her. Finally Richard told Shelly to go and tell the others the bad news. Later, our friend, Dorris, told me that Richard just kept saying over and over again, "They didn't get it all, what are we going to do?" as he paced back and forth in the room.

When I woke up I was being wheeled into recovery and the first thing I said was, "Did they get it all?" The nurse responded with "Well, we took a lot of tissue." From that statement I assumed that we would have to wait for the pathology report, which would probably take at least a day or two. I must have gone right back to sleep because I don't remember being in the recovery room at all. Shelly told me later that I was very, very sick in recovery. When she saw me throwing up, she knew it was bad, because for me throwing up comes right before dying. I do remember being wheeled into an elevator and taken to my room. I was so "in-and-out-of-it" that I don't remember much at all. When Richard and Shelly heard the bad news from the surgeon, they told her that they would prefer that she tell me the situation because they knew that I would have a lot of questions that they would not be able to answer.

The surgeon was not going to be able to see me until the next morning, so they would have to stay with me through the whole night. They were just hoping and praying that I didn't ask the dreaded question, so they would not have to tell me. I don't think Richard could handle it, so he decided to go on home. He left Shelly to stay with me. I was very restless during the night. I noticed that Shelly was being very quiet, and I just thought she probably didn't want to disturb me. Little did I know that she was totally terrified that I would ask her about the surgery.

There was a recliner in the room, so Shelly tried to get some rest, but it was so very uncomfortable. At one point I said to Shelly, "I guess they got it all". It wasn't in the form of a question: it was more like a statement. Shelly didn't say anything in response, and in a few minutes she got up and left the room for a while. I thought that she probably just wanted to get some fresh air. Little did I know that she had gone to her car and, in the quietness and privacy of the night, she sobbed and sobbed until she was finally able to pull herself back together. While she was gone, I managed to fall asleep, so I wasn't aware of how long she was gone. She was in the recliner when I woke up; but she said that she was going next door where she had seen an empty bed and she would try to sleep some. If I needed her, I should just call and she would come. She got a little rest and relief from the tension that she was feeling when she was with me. I did have to call her to come and help me get to the bathroom, and she came running to help. I never did outright ask Shelly if they got all the cancer. I guess I was thinking that we would have to wait for the pathology report, which would probably not come for a few days. Of course Shelly didn't know this, and she could not believe that I wasn't asking questions. She just thought that her prayers were being answered, and in a way they were. The Lord was sparing her from the ordeal of telling me that the surgery was not successful.

GOING HOME

Somehow, we made it through the night and we were just waiting for the surgeon to come so that I could be dismissed to go home. Richard had already made it back to the hospital before dawn. I had been given some pain medication so I was feeling OK. They brought a breakfast tray in for me and I was actually feeling hungry, but when the nurse lifted the cover off the plate, out of nowhere, I just threw up right on top of the food. It was if someone had flipped a switch and it just happened. That is the only time I remember throwing up during the whole time since April 5th. Of course, I had been very sick in recovery, but I do not remember that at all.

When the surgeon finally came in, I didn't even ask *her* if they got it all. She began to explain to me that during the surgery they kept cutting away skin on the lower part of the incision trying to get a clear margin. Finally they had to stop because there was not going to be enough skin left to close the incision, so she was not able to get a clear margin. She said that this had never happened to any of her patients before. I just looked at her and asked her what that meant. She said that she was not able to get all of the cancer. She said since it is not recommended that IBC patients have reconstruction immediately after surgery because of the high risk of recurrence, there was not a plastic surgeon standing by in the operating room. If there had been, then once she achieved clear margins, the plastic surgeon could have stepped in and closed using whatever techniques were needed. I listened to what she said, and a hundred thoughts must have gone through my head. I am a problem solver by nature, and this was definitely a problem. My inclination was to try and solve the problem, but my brain just would not work. Since I could not come up with a single solution, I finally managed to ask her what our next step would be. She said that she would give me about two weeks and then she wanted me to come to her office, and we would do biopsies to find where the margin of cancer was; and then try a re-excision (more surgery in the same incision) to remove all of it. After that was completed, she would call in the plastic surgeon (the one I had gone to for a consultation just in case I was ever eligible for reconstruction). I guessed that this would make me eligible. The plastic surgeon would perform a partial reconstruction using a shoulder-flap from my back to provide enough skin to close the incision. We had a plan for solving the problem, and that is what would keep me going. I was scheduled for a post-op appointment on Wednesday the 23rd, and for the biopsies on Wednesday the 30th. I would just focus on these next steps and trust the Lord for the outcome . . . one step at a time, one day at a time.

The surgeon completed all of the necessary paper work for me to be released from the hospital that day. Then a nurse came in to show us how to "milk" the tube, which was protruding from my right side and my now very flat chest. This procedure would need to be performed several times a day in order to allow any accumulated fluid to pass through the tube and into the soft plastic bulb at the end of the tube. Richard decided that he would wait outside while the nurse gave Shelly and me the instructions. She demonstrated how to put the tube between our forefinger and thumb and pull it down from the chest toward the bulb while holding the tube near the incision. When the bulb became full, we would need to empty it and then reattach it to the tube so more fluid could drain into the bulb. I was fine with all of this, and Shelly and I were trying to pay close attention to the instructions. Everything was going well . . . until the nurse asked Shelly to try it. When Shelly took the tube and began to "milk" it, all of a sudden, she got very dizzy and had to sit down. She was as white as the hospital sheet on the bed. She was not good with needles and tubes and blood. She finally recovered, and the nurse was able to complete the instructions for the tube. She also gave us a diagram of exercises that I should start right away so that I would not loose my range of motion in my right arm. She wanted me to try and touch the inside of my right elbow to my right ear before I left the hospital. The only way I could even come close to doing that was to tilt my head to the right as far as I could, which still didn't touch my arm. I was also given a prescription for pain medication and for nausea; so we would need to go by the pharmacy before going home.

The American Cancer Society presented me with a small gift bag that contained a pillow that I could place under my arm to help relieve some of the pressure that I would be feeling, and also gave me a beautiful white teddy bear with pink ribbons on the bottom of its feet.

Finally, we were allowed to leave the hospital: it had not even been twenty-three hours since I had checked in. I placed the pillow under my arm and I held the teddy bear up against my chest so no one could tell that I didn't have a breast there anymore. We didn't talk much on the way home. I was praying silently, and I know that Richard and Shelly were praying, too. This is not what any of us had expected. We were so looking forward to having all of this behind us, except for the radiation treatments. How could this be happening?

RECOVERING FROM THE SURGERY

During the next week, I managed to work at home some while tending to my incision and my drain tube. Shelly had stayed with me on Friday, Saturday and Sunday after the surgery and helped me with the tube. She was doing much better with the tube than she did in the hospital. She had to go back to teaching on Monday. I wasn't able to wear a bra except for the soft bra-like halter they gave me before leaving the hospital. I had also received a foam breast form to place in the soft bra, but I wasn't ready for anything to touch me yet. I just wore my gown and housecoat with a pocket for the drain bulb to fit in, which was not like me at all. I never wore my PJ's when I worked. I did get to take a shower after the first two days, and that was a welcomed pleasure. The warm water running over my body helped me to relax for the first time since my surgery.

I was finally able to get dressed on the day I was scheduled for my post-op appointment with my surgeon. I even managed to put the foam breast form in my soft halter, but it really didn't feel good at all. My appointment wasn't until 11:00 AM, so at least we wouldn't have to wade through rush hour traffic to get to her office. When we finally were called in to see the surgeon, she removed the clear plastic tape that had covered my incision for a week. There had been some bleeding that had dried so the nurse had to clean all of that away. There were actually no stitches to be removed on the outside, so the surgeon began to remove the steri-strips that were all along the incision.

The healing was progressing very well but there were two small areas that had not yet completely healed. The nurse put new steri-strips back all along the incision to keep it closed while the final areas healed. We talked about the biopsy process that would take place in another week and also about the final pathology report from the surgery. It confirmed what we already knew about not getting clear margins in the skin, but it also revealed something which I was not prepared to hear. The tests showed that nine out of the sixteen lymph nodes that were removed during surgery were positive for malignant cancer cells. I had heard about people who's cancer had spread to the lymph nodes, and I knew that this was not good news. However, this would not alter our plan for a re-excision to try and get clear margins in the skin. I would just focus on that plan for now and turn the rest over to the Lord who is the great physician. We returned home that day a little less optimistic than when we left, but I had to remember to just take one step at a time, one day at a time. In our Methodist Hymnal I had come across a beautiful prayer that could be prayed for people who were very ill. The prayer goes like this:

> "O God, who doest forgive our iniquities and heal our diseases, we cry unto Thee. Our strength has been brought low and we know not what the future holds. In our bodies there is pain, in our souls, anxiety and unrest. If it may be, restore us to health. But, if in the order of nature, our suffering must continue, help us to accept it without rebellion. If it must lead us toward the valley of the shadow, help us to fear no evil, but to go bravely into Thy nearer presence. Into Thy hands we commend our body and our spirit. Do with us as thou wilt. In Jesus name.
>
> Amen"

I had already prayed this many times for other people who were ill and now I found myself praying it for me.

EXPRESSIONS OF LOVE

I was still sending updates to all my family, friends and prayer warriors about all of the events that had taken place. I was so very thankful to all of them during this time. There were so many cards, e-mails and calls from so many people who wanted to express their sincere concern for me, and for my family. My dear friends in our little Birthday Club were so good to me, sending me flowers and bringing dinner over every night for a week after my surgery. My dear housekeeper, who came twice a month, brought me some homemade chicken soup. My Mother made my favorite chicken and dumplings. When I didn't feel like eating anything else, I could always eat her chicken and dumplings. All kinds of my favorite foods were prepared and brought to me. Of course, I liked anything that I didn't have to cook.

One dear, dear friend and pastor's wife belonged to a prayer shawl ministry. They had knitted a prayer shawl just for me so I could wrap it around me and feel the love that went into every stitch and know that they all were praying for my complete recovery. Another pastor's wife, whom I had never even met, who had also been through breast cancer, brought me a comfort blanket made by her prayer group to keep me warm during the long winter nights ahead. Her visit was so inspiring to me. There she was—living proof that you could be completely cured of breast cancer. We talked for a long time. It was so good to have someone who really understood what I was going through.

I got cards from people that I had not seen or heard from in years, and from some people that did not even know me, but were praying for me because someone had asked them to. There were even people praying in other states. I heard from former pastors that had been at our little church. It was so comforting to know that so many people wanted to show their love through their many acts of kindness. I thanked God for all of them everyday, and I asked Him to bless them as He blessed me through them each day. They were living out the commandment to "love one another as I have loved you".

POST CHEMO CHECK-UP

The very next day, I had my one-month follow up appointment with my oncologist. I took my little pillow with me and I would have taken my teddy bear but I was able to wear the foam breast form which helped me to appear almost normal; but somehow I knew that I would never be normal again. My oncologist had already been informed of the situation. She examined the incision and said that it looked very good. I told her that I felt like I had an inner tube under my arm where there was still swelling from the surgery. The little pillow they gave me in the hospital really did help to relieve some of the pressure I was feeling. She told me that it was normal to have that feeling and that, in time, it would go away when the swelling went down.

I also expressed to her that since April 5th up until my last chemotherapy treatment, I had always been involved in some form of treatment for the cancer. It had now been five weeks since I had my last chemo, and during that time I had not been taking any kind of treatment to fight the cancer. The surgery was supposed to be the treatment that would make me cancer free, but it didn't. Now that I still had the disease in my body, I felt like I needed to be taking some kind of treatment or doing something instead of just waiting. My oncologist said that she could understand my concern and that she felt the same way. She said that there was something we could do. She reminded me of the test that had been done in the very beginning, which showed that I was ER/PR positive. That meant that I would be eligible for long term treatment using hormones that the cancer cells were receptive to as part of the post-surgery treatment. Most people who were eligible for this kind of treatment had been prescribed Tamoxifin, which should be taken for five years. This treatment had been successfully used to help in the prevention of a reoccurrence. The new drug of choice for this long term treatment was now Femara and she wanted to start me on it right away. She prepared a prescription so that I could get it on the way home that day. I felt so relieved to know that I would be doing something to fight the cancer instead of just waiting to heal enough so that the biopsies could be done. Now I finally knew why those test results in the very beginning were such good news.

SECOND OPINION

Sometime during the next few days, my sister-in-law, Brenda (Gene's wife), made a suggestion that I might want to get a second opinion to find out what other options were available to me. She suggested that I might try to go to the M. D. Anderson Cancer Center in Houston to see what they would recommend, especially since this situation had never presented itself to my surgeon before. I talked it over with Richard and Shelly and some of my other family members, and they all agreed that it would be a good thing to get a second opinion.

So I began the process by going on the Internet to find out some information about M. D. Anderson Cancer Center. To my surprise, there was a satellite center in Orlando, Florida, which was only about eight hours away by car. There were also links to "consultations" on the website. I called the number listed and informed the person who answered that I was interested in getting a second opinion for my situation. She was very helpful. She assigned me to a doctor and set up an appointment for November 11th (my birthday) at 8:30AM. She gave me instructions on how to get my records to the center and told me what I should bring with me. She gave specific instructions on where to go once we got to the center.

The only thing left for me to do was to call my surgeon and my oncologist and request that they fax or e-mail what records they could and prepare the rest for me to pick up so that I could take them with me. I was a bit anxious about doing this. I did not want them to think that I did not trust them, because I did. I even talked with the psychologist who worked with my oncologist about my fears. She advised me that if a doctor was upset about a patient getting a second opinion I needed to change doctors. Most of the time they welcomed any second opinions.

So I called both doctors' offices and requested that the records be prepared and sent. What I thought would be an impossible task to do in such a short length of time just fell into place. My prayers were answered once again. I kept reminding myself and others that even though things had not turned out as we had hoped, that delay was not denial. I still trusted the Lord and continued to be thankful for each and every day. I had been taking one day at a time for a long time now, and as someone said to me, I should be an expert at it by now. I also remembered the bumblebees that were flying on the day of my first chemotherapy treatment and how they revealed to me that all things are possible with God as our creator. I praised Him for his guidance, protection, comfort and care during this most frightening time.

MARGIN BIOPSY

On Wednesday, October 30th, two weeks since I had my modified radical mastectomy, I returned to my surgeon's office. She planned to take some skin biopsies from the lower edge of the incision in order to determine where the clear margins were located. She started about one inch below the incision and took seven samples. These would be sent to a lab and examined and a written pathology report would follow in about twenty-four to forty-eight hours. Everything went well during the biopsy, so now all we had to do was wait for the report.

WHATEVER HAPPENED TO PHYSICAL THERAPY?

During this same visit, my surgeon referred me to a physical therapist who would be able to help me with the rehabilitation of my right arm. At home I should have been doing more therapy, which was diagramed in the brochure they gave to me before I was discharged from the hospital. With all the flurry of activity since my surgery and after finding out that I still had the cancer, I guess you might say that I had a little set back. My range of movement had declined quite a bit in my right arm following the surgery. If I waited too long after the biopsies to start rehabilitation, I might not ever regain a full range of motion. We were able to make an appointment for the very next day, which was Thursday, October 31st. Also, I needed to have a consultation with a radiologist in order to schedule thirty-five radiation treatments that would start as soon as I healed from the surgery. We were able to set up an appointment for Friday, November 1st. These two things would certainly keep me busy and keep my mind off the biopsy results, which we were anxiously awaiting.

The next day, which was Halloween and the last day of October, I drove to Northside Hospital for my appointment with the physical therapist. Of course, all of the new patient information had to be completed before we could begin. I was given instructions on how to do certain movements and exercises that would help to loosen the tightened muscles and restore a full range of motion to my arm. It was not fun trying to raise my arm so that the inside of my elbow could touch my ear. Each time I would raise my arm I would try to bring it a little closer to my ear without moving my head. With these stretches, if I did them faithfully, I would be able to reach my goal in a few sessions. The therapist showed me how to continue to do them everyday at home. She suggested that I take some Tylenol about thirty minutes before my stretches in order to reduce some of the pain that I was experiencing.

As I returned home, I could not help feeling relief that this month was finally over. I had my surgery as well as the biopsies behind me. As soon as the results came back we would be able to focus on what the next step would be. I praised God for being with us and getting us through these previous seven months. I prayed silently for inner strength and for physical strength. I knew I would be depending on Him to continue to sustain us during the days ahead . . . .

CHAPTER SIX

THE MONTH OF NOVEMBER

HAPPY BIRTHDAY!

The following day, which was Friday, November 1st, I went back to Northside Hospital to meet with my radiologist. He was so very nice and I had heard that he was one of the best in his field. But he only worked out of the Northside Office so if I wanted to have him perform the radiation treatments, I would have to drive everyday to Northside, take my treatment, and then drive back home. With the traffic situation the way it was, I knew this would take at least four hours from the time I left home each day until I returned. This would mean that I would have thirty five four hour sessions lasting seven weeks. After we met with the radiologist, I talked it over with Richard and we both decided it would be better to find someone that could provide the treatments at the Alpharetta location. I called my oncologist to see if she could refer me to someone in her building or in the complex that could administer the radiation treatments. She did know of an excellent radiologist, and we were able to schedule a consultation for Tuesday, November 26th. We also learned that the Alpharetta office had the same kind of equipment that was used at the Northside location.

The afternoon of this same day, my surgeon called to let me know the results of the biopsies taken to determine how far we would have to go to get clear margins in the skin. She told me that all of the samples had come back negative! So all we needed to do was take off no more than another inch and have the plastic surgeon perform the partial shoulder flap reconstruction to close the incision! This would make me pathologically cancer free before going on to radiation therapy. We were all so relieved and so excited to hear this good news! I praised God for such a great report! The re-excision was scheduled for Wednesday, November 13th, which wasn't nearly soon enough as far as I was concerned.

We all were so very happy to once again have a plan on which we could focus. I didn't have anything scheduled until Friday, November 8th, which was another session with the physical therapist. I would have seven days without seeing any kind of doctor or nurse or needle. This would give me some time to catch up on some work in my office and maybe have a little time to regroup. We had all been on an emotional roller coaster for the last five or six weeks. We all needed to reflect on what had taken place and prepare ourselves for what lay ahead. I was still praising God for all that had been accomplished and for all that would be accomplished, and for sustaining us each day.

On Friday, November 8th, I attended my second physical therapy session. The therapist was very impressed with the progress that I had made. She introduced some more vigorous exercises for me to add to my physical therapy routine. I was surprised that I was able to do most of them without too much pain. Of course, I had remembered to take some Tylenol before I left home.

I also had been scheduled for a pre-surgery consultation with the plastic surgeon on that same day. I was able to go directly from my physical therapy session to her office. While I was there she explained in detail what would take place once my surgeon was able to confirm that clear margins had been obtained. She made me feel confidant that all of the procedures could be accomplished and that I could be pathologically free of cancer when the surgery was completed. That was a comforting thought for me to carry with me that day.

On Saturday night, November 9th, I began packing to leave for the MD Anderson Cancer Center in Orlando, Florida. We planned to leave the next morning so we could spend the night at a hotel and hopefully get some sleep. We would be ready for our early morning appointment with the oncologist who was to review my case and give a second opinion about the procedures that had been planned and explain any other options that might be possible. We planned to return on Monday if possible, but no later than Tuesday, since my re-excision would be on Wednesday.

A wise man once said, "Whatever came to me, I looked on as God's gift for some special purpose. If it was a difficulty, then I knew He had given it to me to struggle with in order to strengthen my mind and my faith." This idea has sweetened my life, and will continue to help me for the rest of my life. I am reminded of the story in the Bible of Joseph and the coat of many colors.

In reading it, one might think that Joseph was the unluckiest person in the universe and was born to loose. It seemed that everywhere he turned calamity greeted him. But God, in His infinite wisdom, was preparing him for the most incredible task of saving His people. In the process Joseph was able to forgive his brothers and was reunited with his entire family. Joseph never lost his faith in God, but continued to trust Him at every turn. He knew what I, too, have come to know, that "In Thy good keeping, all is well."

Our trip to Orlando was uneventful. We arrived in late afternoon and checked into the hotel where we had managed to get a reservation. It was very near the M. D. Anderson Cancer Center. The next day would be my 56th birthday, so we decided to celebrate early. We asked the desk clerk if he could recommend a nice restaurant in the area where we could celebrate, and he directed us to one nearby. We had a very nice dinner and came back to our room and rested from the day of travel before retiring for the night. Our appointment was at 8:30 AM, so we planned to leave early in case we had any difficulty in finding the doctor's office where the appointment was scheduled.

I don't think either one of us got very much sleep that night, so we were both glad when the alarm finally went off. Richard wished me a Happy Birthday with a kiss and we both got up to face the day. The directions we received were very good so we didn't have any trouble at all finding the right place. We arrived about an hour before my appointment but we didn't care. We just stayed in the waiting room and read every magazine and newspaper there.

When I was finally called, Richard and I were ushered to an examination room where I was instructed to undress from the waist up and put the paper gown on with the opening in the front instead of the back. Of course, I already knew how this was done since this would be about the 100th time I had been examined. The oncologist was very thorough and kind. She had reviewed all of the reports and test results that she had received and was very knowledgeable about my situation. She also took the files that I had brought with me. She asked me a lot of questions in order to get as much information as she could so that she could give an informed opinion. After the exam was over she said she wanted some time to review the material that we had brought with us, and then she would give us her opinion. I got dressed and we were sent to a different waiting room.

After some time, we were called back and she sat us both down and began to give us her opinion. She had reviewed the information that I had given her and she had contacted two other physicians in Houston and discussed my case with them. One of the first things she said was that all of the test results that she had seen revealed that I was ER/PR negative, but that my oncologist and I must be under the impression that I was ER/PR positive or I wouldn't be taking

Femara. I told her that I *was* ER/PR positive, but she explained to me that the test did not show that. She pulled out the report and showed me where it had a negative result! I just couldn't believe it!! The only good news that I had gotten in the very beginning wasn't even true! She suggested that I discontinue the Femara but assured me that there were no harmful results from taking it.

The doctor went on to say that I still had a lot of disease left at the time of surgery, even after taking four AC treatments and four Taxotere treatments I still had a 2.5 cm tumor remaining to be removed. She did recommend that we try to obtain clear margins by re-excision as suggested by my surgeon, and that in addition to the thirty-five radiation treatments that had been prescribed, I should also have twelve more chemotherapy treatments of Taxol along with Herceptin to be administered once a week for twelve weeks in conjunction with the radiation; and that Herceptin should be continued for a period of one year. She did say that the radiologist may not want me to take Herceptin along with the radiation and, if that were the case, I should wait until after the radiation treatments were finished to start the Herceptin treatments. She informed me that the results of the pathology report from the surgery had revealed that the cancer had metastasized to eleven or twelve lymph nodes, more than was stated in the original report. She recommended that I have a full body CT Scan with dye to check for any other areas of disease. She said that it was almost 100% certain that the cancer would return even if I followed all of the recommendations in this opinion. She stated that she would follow up with a written report to my oncologist. She asked me if I understood all that we had discussed, and I told her that I did and that I would follow up with my oncologist when I returned home. Happy Birthday to me!

HERCEPTIN

When the doctor at M. D. Anderson Cancer Center suggested that my treatment after surgery should include the drug Herceptin, that was not the first time I had heard about this drug. I had met at least two people in the chemo lab who were taking Herceptin treatments. Their breast cancer had metastasized to another area of their body and there was nothing else that could be done that would produce a cure for their cancer. The Herceptin treatments were part of a clinical trial for women whose cancer had spread to other areas to see if the Herceptin would keep it at bay so they could lead fairly normal lives with cancer. It is similar to a person who has Kidney failure. There is no cure; but dialysis can keep them alive for several years, and they can still maintain a somewhat normal lifestyle. I had talked to my oncologist about this drug earlier and she had informed me then that I was not eligible to be included in the clinical trials since there was no evidence that my cancer had spread to other areas. With this in mind and with the doctor's suggestion that I have a full body CT Scan when I returned home, I imagined that she was almost certain that the cancer had already invaded another area of my body. I determined right then and there that I would not think about that possibility until it was proven to me that the cancer had spread. I just tucked that idea in my little basket along with all the other "goodies" the doctor had delivered to me for my birthday that day.

GOING HOME, AGAIN

We gathered all our belongings that we had brought with us and started the long trip back home. We didn't talk much on the way. We just wanted to be together and not think about the outside world right then. It was just Richard and me taking a trip together, enjoying the sites and silently making memories for another time, another day.

It was late in the afternoon when I suddenly remembered that I had an appointment to make a call to Northside Hospital for pre-registration for surgery on Wednesday, November 13th. I grabbed my cell phone and dialed the number that I had written down in my pocket calendar, but nothing happened. I could not get a signal for my phone, so I waited a few minutes and tried again but still no signal. Finally, I realized my phone's battery was very low, so we decided to stop somewhere and use my calling card to make the call. The appointed time for me to make the call had already passed, but I thought that I would still try to make the call. We stopped at a local Comfort Inn in the town of Forsyth, Georgia. I explained the situation to the front desk clerk and she was so very nice and cooperative about letting me use her phone to place a long distance call using my calling card. I finally got through to the hospital, but since my appointment time had passed the person said that she would have to call me back after her next call. I gave her the number of the motel so she could call me back. We waited about fifteen or twenty minutes in the lobby where the clerk had arranged for a phone to be placed so I would be able to talk from there if the call came in for me. The phone finally rang and it was the call I was expecting. I was able to complete the pre-registration, which confirmed that I would be having the re-excision surgery on Wednesday, November 13th.

We got home late that night and we were both so exhausted. Driving for eighteen hours in three days was worse than digging ditches, and I didn't even do any of the driving. I know Richard was really wiped out. We tried to get some rest so we would be able to work some on Tuesday before my surgery on Wednesday.

RE-EXCISION

I was scheduled for the re-excision at 1:00 PM, so I was not able to eat or drink anything that morning. Even though I wanted this surgery to be over, I was still nervous about it. We left for the hospital in plenty of time to be there for the final registration procedures. Once again, Richard and Shelly were able to be with me right up to the time I was taken to surgery. My mother and sisters had also come to be there for support. This procedure was not scheduled to be outpatient surgery due to the fact that I was scheduled for two separate surgeries. My surgeon had informed me that I might be in the hospital a few days depending on how I was doing after the partial flap reconstruction.

Before the surgery began, and after talking with me, the surgeon and the plastic surgeon spoke with Richard and Shelly in the surgery waiting room. They informed them of the length of time it would take to perform both surgeries and that they would be given updates along the way. Shelly had a request to make to the plastic surgeon. She asked her if, when she was taking the flap section from my shoulder, she could also remove this ugly mole between my shoulder blades. The plastic surgeon just laughed and said, "Oh no, we can save that for the nipple later!" Then they all had a good laugh.

I woke up in recovery and it felt like *de ja vu*. I had the same clear plastic bandage and the same drain tube protruding from the side of my chest. I wondered if I was having a bad dream. My first question to ask was, "Did they get it all?" and with big smiles Richard and Shelly both assured me that they had. Even better, they did not have to do the partial reconstructive surgery. Apparently the plastic surgeon was able to perform some "skin stretching" and they were able to close without using the shoulder flap section of skin. This was all wonderful news. **I was overjoyed to be pathologically cancer free!** I would be able to go home in the morning and start my recovery once again, then on to radiation and more chemotherapy.

I was dismissed from the hospital the next morning on the orders of my surgeon. I did not see the plastic surgeon before I left. I was however scheduled to see her on the following Tuesday, November 19th at 10:45AM for a post-surgery check-up, and I was also scheduled to see my surgeon immediately after my appointment with the plastic surgeon for another post-surgery check-up.

RECOVERING ONCE AGAIN

I spent the next few days resting as much as possible and taking care of my 'milking duties' with the drain. I didn't even try to go downstairs to work until the following Monday. Even then I was still feeling very weak and drained of energy. I attempted to do some work and managed to get a few things off my desk that were priority issues. Once again my dear friends and family were bringing food and helping me with laundry and other chores. I was so thankful to have them helping. I really was becoming weary of all we had been through. In spite of having the incision in the same exact site as before, my healing was progressing very well.

POST-OP FOLLOW UPS

By Tuesday, I was able to get dressed with all of the accoutrements necessary to appear normal. We were to see the plastic surgeon first, since she was the one who had placed the drain tube. We arrived early, as usual, and waited the usual period of time and read the usual magazines and various other papers and books that were there for that purpose. I had kept the log showing how much fluid had been draining into the bulb at the end of the tube. There had been hardly any during this day, so when the doctor saw the log she instructed the nurse to remove the drain tube, which she proceeded to do. After removing the tube, she placed a square piece of gauze affixed with surgical tape to cover the hole where the tube had been. The plastic surgeon examined me and said that I was healing very well. Unless I had any other problems, I could be dismissed from her care and continue to see my surgeon for any follow-up visits that were needed.

We left there and went to a nearby restaurant to get a bite to eat before it was time for my appointment with my surgeon. We arrived early for my appointment. As I signed in I could see that it was going to be a long afternoon because the first waiting room was almost full. Finally, I was called back to the second waiting room and I changed into my blue robe and took my place with all of the other ladies waiting for their turn. As I sat there I began to feel something running down my side. I placed my hand into my robe and discovered that there was a reddish fluid dripping from the bandage. I was able to get the attention of my surgeon's nurse and she took me back to a room where she changed the bandage so I wouldn't bleed all over the waiting room floor. She sent me back out to the waiting room until the doctor was available to see me for the follow-up examination. I sat in the waiting room for a while and once again I felt that uncomfortable feeling of something running down my side. I was also beginning to feel a lot of pain near the hole where the tube had been. Before I could get the nurse's attention, I heard them call my name. I was very relieved to be going to a room where I could lay down for awhile.

When the doctor came in I explained to her that I was apparently still having some drainage and that I had already soaked two bandages with a bloodlike fluid. She immediately determined that the drain tube had been taken out too soon and she informed me that she was going to make a small incision near my breastbone and allow the fluid that was building up in my chest cavity to drain out. I was instructed to hold a stack of gauze bandages over the incision and to apply pressure for about forty-five minutes in order to absorb most of the fluid. She then would be able to make a "rubber glove" drain at that site so I would be able to go home. I was moved to another room where I was given a local shot to numb the area and the incision was made. There was a lot of blood at first, but she assured me that it was OK. So, for the next forty-five minutes, I held pressure on the spot but the stack of gauze kept getting soaked with blood, so I had to have the nurse give me a new stack of gauze several times to use to apply the pressure.

The pain was gradually getting worse and worse and I was becoming more and more uncomfortable. I asked the nurse if I could have something for the pain, and she said she would check with the doctor. When the surgeon came in, she looked at me and could tell I was in a lot of pain. She also looked at the used stacks of gauze, which were soaked with blood. She quickly examined me once again and determined that it was not fluid that was building up in my chest cavity, it was actually blood. She said that there must be a hematoma somewhere. I asked: "What is a hematoma?" She explained that there was blood leaking from an artery and that unfortunately the only way to stop it required emergency surgery! I could not believe what I was hearing! I can't have surgery again, not in this same place! It hurts too much for anyone to touch it right now! She said that she did not have anything for pain in the office but she would send someone to the pharmacy across the street to get a prescription for some pain medication.

By now, the nurse had gone to get my husband to let him know what was happening. I told him that I had some Tylenol in my purse and to give it to me now. As soon as he did, the doctor sent him across the street to get the pain medication. He hurried as fast as he could. He was so upset that he got very impatient and angry with the pharmacist who was not moving fast enough to fill the prescription. He came running back with the pills and I took two right away.

The doctor had decided that it would be better if I could get to my car and let Richard drive me to the Emergency Room at Northside Hospital, which was only a block away. If not we would have to wait for an ambulance to come and take me to the hospital. I said that I thought I could make it to the car. The nurse helped me up and I just wrapped the robe around me and she helped me walk toward the exit. Richard had already left to get the car. By the time we got to the sidewalk, Richard was waiting for me and was able to help me into the car. I was trying so very hard to stay conscience, but it was getting very difficult. The pain was getting very intense and I was crying, not only from the pain, but from the whole situation. This can't be happening! I have not even healed from the last surgery and they are going to rip it open again! Richard drove as fast as he could to the emergency room, which had been alerted to the fact that we were on our way.

There was a wheelchair waiting for me and I was rushed into the emergency room where we would fill out paper work. We were just waiting for my surgeon to arrive. She said she would quickly alert her remaining patients about the situation and get to the hospital as soon as possible to get prepped for surgery. Richard had managed to call my sister, Marilyn, to let her know what was happening and asked her to let the rest of the family know. Her daughter, Susan lived near by, and Marilyn had called her first, so she came in shortly after we arrived. I asked her to please help me get to the restroom. She rolled me as far as she could and then helped me out of the wheelchair. I literally screamed from the pain. I apologized to her, but I told her that I was in so much pain. She said to just go ahead and scream if I needed to.

EMERGENCY SURGERY

As soon as Susan and I got back to the area where we had been waiting, they said that they were ready for me to go in for the surgery. Shelly had just arrived and we only had a few minutes before they started an IV. It didn't take long before I was beginning to feel the effects of the medication. Then, before I knew it, I was saying goodbye to Richard and Shelly and Susan and they said they were praying for me and told me to behave myself and get back as soon as possible. So here I was, being rolled into the operating room once again. I was just praying that they would be able to fix whatever was wrong and that everything would be OK. I just placed myself in God's hands once again and trusted Him for the outcome.

The surgery lasted for about an hour and I was in recovery for about an hour. When I woke up, Richard and Shelly were there with me. The surgeon had met with them and told them what had happened. Apparently when the drain tube was removed at the plastic surgeon's office somehow it sucked a hole right out of an artery and every time my heart would beat it was pumping blood into my chest cavity. She said that she literally had to "mop me out" and that I had lost about a pint of blood. She said if the artery had been severed it would have recoiled and healed itself; but it just had a gaping hole in it and the blood was just leaking out and going everywhere. Thankfully she was able to repair the artery and stop the loss of blood just in time. She had to put another drain tube in to allow the fluid to drain from the incision. I truly know that the Lord was surely watching over me. I shutter to think what would have happened if I had not had the follow-up appointment with my surgeon.

Once again I spent the night in the hospital. This time Richard stayed with me, because Shelly had to go back to school the next day. I had a very restless night, and so did Richard. I was feeling very weak and Richard said I was as pale as a ghost. I was able to eat something that morning without throwing up, so I was allowed to go home. The nurse began to show me how to clear the tube of any fluid, but I told her that this was my third drain tube in less than five weeks and it wouldn't be necessary to demonstrate the procedure. We were given the usual instructions about how to care for the incision and I was scheduled for a follow-up appointment in a week. I was also given a prescription for pain medication to use, as needed. I was wheeled out to the patient pick-up area where Richard was waiting in the car. He got out and helped me get into the car because he could see that I was still very weak.

FOLLOW UP WITH ONCOLOGIST

We started home and I remembered that I had an appointment with my oncologist. If we drove straight there, we would be right on time for my appointment. Richard drove to the front door of the building and helped me out of the car and to a bench, which was right at the front door, and he told me to sit right there until he could park the car. The pain medication that they had administered before I left the hospital was helping to thwart the pain, but it was making me feel very woozy. I managed to keep my composure while Richard parked the car.

We entered the oncologist's office with Richard holding onto me to keep me upright. He sat me down and registered for me at the desk. We were called in right away because they already knew that I had been in the hospital for the emergency surgery. I was able to talk with my oncologist about all of the things I had learned from the oncologist at the M. D. Anderson Cancer Center, even the part about the 100% chance that it would come back. The last thing we talked about was the ER/PR test results. She said she would have to study my records and review the test once more before she could confirm what had been stated in the second opinion, which she had already received from the oncologist at the M. D. Anderson Cancer Center. I told her that I had already taken myself off the Femara and she said that was OK for now and not to worry about it. She said that I should go home and get some rest, and as soon as I would be able, we would talk about scheduling for the weekly chemotherapy treatments of Taxol. She also told me once again, that as long as there was no evidence of metastasis the federal guidelines did not allow me to be treated with Herceptin at this time. However, she had already scheduled me for a full CT Scan as recommended in the written opinion. It was set up for Tuesday, November 26th, which would be the following Tuesday, two days before Thanksgiving. We got home and I went straight to bed. I was totally exhausted. I slept for the rest of the day and night, getting up only to eat some soup for dinner.

POST EMERGENCY OP FOLLOW UP

I did not even try to go downstairs to do any work until the following Monday, which was November 25th. Even then, I still felt like my strength was not coming back, and I was wondering if I would ever feel better again. My follow up visit with my surgeon was scheduled for 3:00 PM on this same day, and I tried to work as much as I could up until the time for us to leave for the appointment.

We arrived at her office and I was still experiencing the weakness. Richard registered me at the front desk and before long they called me back to the second waiting room where I changed into my blue robe once more. I didn't have long to wait before they put me in a room where I could lay down and wait for the doctor. She came in and asked me how in the world I was doing and I told her that I really wasn't feeling that great. She said she could certainly understand. She examined the incision and instructed the nurse to take out the drain tube. I tried not to panic at the thought of this so I began to pray that everything would be OK. The nurse was in the process of training a new person and as she was removing the tube, I heard her stress the fact that she must always let the pressure out of the bulb before removing the tube. That's when I realized what had happened at the plastic surgeon's office. Apparently the nurse had not released the pressure on the bulb, and that's what caused the hole to be sucked out of the artery!

The surgeon came back in and talked with me about everything that had happened. She said she had called my plastic surgeon after the emergency surgery and informed her about what had taken place. The plastic surgeon said that had never happened to any of her patients before. When she told me that, I remembered that was the same thing that my surgeon had said when she was not able to remove all of the cancer during the first operation. It seemed to me that this situation was happening to me a lot more than I cared for. My surgeon said that she would have called the plastic surgeon beforehand and let her do the surgery, but there wasn't any time to waste. I had already lost about a pint of blood so the surgery had to be done as soon as possible.

I was so thankful that everything had worked out OK. I was glad that she had been there and that somehow I was in the right place at just the right time. I knew that divine intervention was at work in my life once again. I continue to be amazed at God's planning and timing. What I don't understand is why He was always there watching over me and protecting me. I am humbled and grateful for answered prayers and for His daily provision. He has continued to sustain me through all of these trials. What a great and awesome God is He!!

NO REST FOR THE WEARY!

Before we left the surgeon's office I picked up all of the films of my mammograms that the surgeon had in my files. I was to take them with me to the radiologist for her to review during my first consultation with her, which was scheduled for 1:00 PM the following day, Tuesday, November 26th. My oncologist had also arranged for me to have a full CT Scan and Echo Cardiogram at Northside Hospital at 8:30AM on the morning of this same day. So I had a full day ahead of me, and I was still feeling very tired and dragged out.

We got up very early the next morning and left the house by 6:30 AM in order to miss the rush hour traffic, and of course we arrived very early at the hospital. I was not allowed to eat anything, which did not help me in the process of trying to gain back my strength. I had to register as an outpatient because of my allergy to iodine, which was used in the CT Scan. I had remembered to take the pre-medication to prevent any reaction during the scan. I was taken for the Echo Cardiogram first. This would help both my oncologist and my new radiologist in determining whether or not I was still physically able to withstand the radiation and the chemotherapy.

After completing this test, we were sent to the outpatient surgery waiting room to wait to be called for the CT Scan. It was finally my turn, so I was ushered to one of the spaces that was separated only by curtains from the persons on either side, who were also outpatients. I undressed completely and put on the cotton gown which could be opened at the back this time. I brought some socks with me because my feet would always get so cold. The process started with the nurse inserting an IV needle into my left arm. Since having my mastectomy, my right arm was not eligible for needle sticks or blood pressure cuffs, which might cause lymphodema in that arm. The nurse started the procedure and after probing my arm for several minutes, he decided to try another spot. Once again he was not able to get a vein. He said that he was only permitted to try two times to insert the needle, and then he would yield to another person. So he called another IV nurse to try and get a good vein. After two tries, she was not able to find anything either. I apparently was very dehydrated. I had forgotten to drink lots of water the day before, which would have helped greatly in this process. The second nurse told me that she was going to have to call the Head IV Nurse. Well, I thought, I guess you learn something new everyday. I didn't know hospitals even had a Head IV Nurse.

There were about five people in the room by this time. Some were the technicians who operated the CT machine and two of them were the nurses who had been working on my arm. Someone made the call and said that it would be about fifteen minutes before the Head IV Nurse could come. They suggested that I get up and walk around which would help to relieve some of the tension that I was feeling. When I got up, you could see the outline of my body on the sheet where I had sweated and there was also some blood that had stained the sheet. I walked around for a few minutes, and when I got back, I asked if there was anyone there who was a praying person—if so, would they please pray for me. They said they already were. That was so very comforting to me. I immediately felt the tension melt away.

I started to lay back down and I noticed that someone had changed the sheets. They had even warmed them so the sheets wouldn't feel cold to me. The Head IV Nurse arrived; and when I laid down I told everyone that those old sheets were the problem, and these new ones were going to make all the difference. They all laughed as the nurse started her probe. She got it on the first try! She just looked at me and said "I guess it must have been the sheets after all!" We all laughed again. Thank goodness our prayers were answered! The rest of the test was uneventful, and I was certainly thankful for that.

After the test was complete, I got dressed and went back out to where Richard was waiting for me. He was very concerned that I had been gone so long. As we found our way to the cafeteria, I told him what all had happened. I was very hungry and was able to eat a very good breakfast. By the time I finished eating I was feeling much better, and I felt that I had finally started to gain a little strength back.

RADIATION, HERE I COME

We returned home and I was able to rest for about an hour before we had to leave for my appointment with the radiologist. I took the mammograms with me as we started out the door. The consultation was more involved than I had expected. I met with the oncology radiologist (what a mouthful) and she began to explain the procedure that would take place today. There would be a team that would be with me throughout the thirty-five treatments. This team, along with the radiologist, would review the mammograms and the instructions from my oncologist as to exactly where the radiation should be directed.

I was taken to the dressing room where an attendant assigned a robe that I would be using each time I came. My name was taped to the sleeve of the robe so no one else could use it. Once I finished undressing from the waist up and had my gown on, I was taken to the area where the process of "marking" the area for treatment was done. First, I was asked to lie down on a table and raise my right arm up over my head and hold it there while pictures were taken of the area of my chest where the cancer had been. This was a very uncomfortable position even though I had been doing the physical therapy to improve my range of movement. I was instructed that it was very important that I maintain this position for the entire time of this procedure. I told them I didn't think I could do it. I was getting cramps in my side and back and I needed to sit up in order to relieve the cramp. They helped me to sit up and the cramps subsided. Once again, they wanted me to lie down and raise my hand over my head. This time they placed a foam-lined plastic form above my head in which my arm could rest. This helped to relieve the tension and pain I was feeling in the area of the incision. Finally, I got into a position that was a little more comfortable—one I thought I could maintain for an extended period of time.

The technicians began to use a red marking pen to outline the area designated for treatment. It would be very important that the radiation was aimed at the exact location each time. If not, some areas could be under radiated or over radiated. This procedure involved taking measurements with high-tech equipment as well as using a tool manually to confirm the prescribed area of radiation. By the time they finished, I felt like my arm was going to fall off. I had red markings that covered about one fourth of my upper right body. They had placed clear plastic tape over the red markings so they would not be washed away while taking a shower.

I was glad finally to be out from under the scrutinizing eyes of the technicians who were trying desperately, it seemed, to be very concise in making the marks exactly where they were supposed to be. At one point I remember feeling as if I had been kidnapped by aliens who were examining me as a specimen. However, all of the technicians were very kind and very respectful of my modesty. You would think by now, after all I had been through, that I would be over any feelings of modesty; but I still couldn't get use to baring my body to strangers. I was now ready to begin the radiation treatments. I was scheduled for my first one on Thursday, December 5th at 12:00 PM.

THANKSGIVING

Thanksgiving was always a time for our families to be together for good food and fellowship. Everyone always made a special effort to be there. We had Thursday lunch at Richard's Mother's house, and then we visited with my Mother and Dad and brothers and sisters in the afternoon. We planned a get together on Saturday for another Thanksgiving lunch with my family. As usual, I ate too much on both occasions, but it was good to be with family and friends. My sisters and I always go shopping together on the Friday after Thanksgiving, but this year I had to bow out. I was conserving my energy as much as possible for the journey ahead.

Truly this was a year for giving thanks for all the blessings that we have received. Of course, we always think of the blessing of food at Thanksgiving; but there are so many things to thank God for on this day—I am thankful for Richard and Shelly, to have a family close by to support me, to have friends and prayer warriors who express their care and concern in so many ways, for doctors and nurses, for scientific breakthroughs in medicine everyday, to have clothing and shelter, to be near loved ones, to live in the United States and have the freedoms that we enjoy such as worshipping as we choose, voting, the freedom of speech, a justice system designed to protect the innocent and punish the guilty, our parents who taught us right from wrong, our teachers and those who have influenced our lives along the way, our health, and most of all for Jesus Christ who provides a way for salvation to everyone who believes. I am thankful, too, for the sustaining power of the Holy Spirit and the blanket of love and protection He has provided during the second most difficult time in my life. I am also thankful for the promise that I will once again see my beautiful daughter, Lynn, when I get to heaven. It was indeed a time to celebrate!

CHAPTER SEVEN

THE MONTH OF DECEMBER

HAPPY BIRTHDAY, JESUS

December is the beginning of my favorite time of the year. I love the festivities and all the special ways we celebrate the birth of Jesus. Having children, and seeing them learn the importance of this Holiday is one of the greatest gifts in life. This year it would really be hectic with all of the treatments that would be necessary; but still, I looked forward to another Christmas, and I was thankful that I was still here to celebrate with my family and friends.

Once we all recovered from the festivities of Thanksgiving, it was time to get back to the business at hand. I had not had any appointments since my consultation with the radiologist, and that was truly a blessing. On Monday, December 2nd, I had another session with the physical therapist. This would be my first session since the emergency surgery on November 19th. It was like I was starting all over again, so we took it slow at first. I told her that I would be starting my third round of chemotherapy on Wednesday, December 4th, and radiation treatments would begin the following day. We only scheduled two more sessions for the remainder of the month. The next one would be on Monday, December 16th and the final one would be on the following Monday, December 23rd. My assignment was to do the therapy exercises faithfully everyday to reclaim all of my range of motion and also to prevent lymphodema (swelling of the arm which can be caused by lymph node removal).

On Wednesday, December 4th, we once again made the short trek to my oncologist's office to begin the Taxol treatments that had been prescribed by the doctor at M. D. Anderson Cancer Center. Since I had no evidence of metastatic disease, I would not be taking the Herceptin (as had originally been recommended) but would just be taking the Taxol. I had tolerated all of the previous treatments and the surgeries fairly well. I know that the prayers and the support I received from my family, friends and prayer warriors had enabled me to make it through the difficult times of the last eight months. Once again I asked all of them for their continued prayers. I have learned to take one day at a time, and I was thankful for being able to maintain somewhat of a normal daily routine. I depended upon the Lord to give me strength for each day. I learned that I could not think of all the treatments together; I had to just think about today's treatment and get through it. Then I could think about the next day.

When we arrived, I waited for my name to be called. I knew the routine all too well by now. My first stop was at the lab, where I had the usual needle-stick in the left arm for the blood test to see if my counts were good enough to have the treatment. Since the mastectomy and because I had had lymph nodes removed, I could not have any needle-punctures or blood pressure checks on my right arm since that could cause lymphodema. Fortunately, the blood test was good and everything was good to go. My oncologist talked with me about the drugs that I would be taking. I would be given a pre-medication of Decadron to prevent any allergic reaction to the Taxol. The treatments would not be as harsh as the first two rounds, but there could be side effects, which might include nausea and loss of hair; but hopefully these treatments would not wipe out my white and red blood cells, so that was good news to hear. With all the preliminaries out of the way, it was time to get started with the treatment. Everything went according to plans and we were finished in about an hour. Just think, only eleven more to go after this one! Only eleven more weeks and I would have the chemo behind me!

The very next day, we reported to the same medical complex, but to a different building, for my first radiation treatment. The technician said that the scheduled time of 12:00 Noon would be the same for all thirty-five treatments unless their schedule would not allow it for some reason. This was the time that the radiation equipment would be reserved for me. When we arrived I was immediately taken back to the area where the "marking" had taken place. After reviewing the readings, the radiologist had some changes that needed to be made. We went through the intense procedure of positioning my body and arm precisely the right way at the right angles. New marks were made and new tape attached. Once that was completed, it was time to begin the first treatment. I was moved to another room and instructed to lie down on a padded table, which had a huge round machine overhead. We spent some time getting my position on the table exactly and precisely correct for the radiation to be aimed inside the markings. I would be asked to assume this position on the table for each treatment. It required that I keep my arm up over my head during the procedure. I realized that I wouldn't have any trouble maintaining my range of movement after thirty-five days of this kind of stretching. It was very uncomfortable to stay in the position for the treatments on this first day. I was hoping that it would get easier in the days ahead.

The next few weeks proved to be very exhausting. I was trying to work everyday, going to my radiation treatments everyday, and on Wednesday I would have both a chemo treatment and a radiation treatment. Wednesday, December 11th was especially difficult. I had a chemotherapy treatment at 9:00 AM and I had a Christmas luncheon at 12:00 Noon with my employer and co-workers. Because of the luncheon, the radiation lab allowed me to change my schedule so I wouldn't have to be back there until 4:30 PM for my radiation treatment.

It was as if the days just zipped by with so many things going on at once. I was tolerating the radiation fairly well but I have very fair skin and unfortunately it does not hold up well under radiation. By the end of December, I had completed three weeks of radiation and four chemotherapy treatments. I had burns over about one fourth of my upper body, and we were treating them with whatever creams and ointments were prescribed for the week. I even tried pure aloe from the plant, which my very good friend, Renee had given me. These topical solutions relieved the pain a little, but it still felt like a very, very bad sunburn. I was told that I would begin to feel fatigue after about three weeks of radiation and they were right. Of course, I am sure the hectic schedule added to the fatigue. I was still keeping up with my physical therapy each day for my right arm and shoulder. I was trying to attend all of the various special events during this time, and there was also shopping and baking to get done. I am a member of a Birthday Club, and each month we celebrate a member's birthday by going out to dinner with "just the girls". We had been doing this ever since I could remember. In December we would have a "Happy Birthday, Jesus" party at one of our homes. It was always a very special time, especially this year. All of my friends in this little group had been praying for me and cooking and helping in any way they could. I was so thankful for each and every one of them for being in my life.

Other than the radiation burns, I was not having any other side effects. I understand that some people have nausea and vomiting with radiation, but I had been spared so far. The chemo treatments were on every Wednesday.

The radiation lab very kindly arranged for me to come directly there after my chemotherapy, and they would let me take the radiation treatment no matter what time it was. I was very thankful for that. Since my chemo dose was smaller than the ones I had earlier, I was much better able to tolerate it this time. I was not taking any medications for side effects other than some Tylenol and the pre-medications to prevent any allergic reaction to the chemo. My blood counts were not getting wiped out with each treatment; therefore it wasn't necessary for me to take shots to boost my blood cell levels. I didn't even have to take any nausea medication. I was praising the Lord for all of these good things. About the only side effects for me were the loss of my normal taste of food for three to four days after chemo and, oh yes, my hair which was just starting to grow back was falling out again. Like Richard once said, hair was highly over rated anyway. We would listen to the lyrics of the song "Forever and Ever Amen" by Randy Travis that says "They say time takes it's toll on a body, makes a young girls brown hair turn gray. Well, honey I don't care, I ain't in love with your hair and if it all fell out I'd love you anyway."

Before I knew it, it was Tuesday, December 24th, Christmas Eve. The radiation lab requested that all patients come in early that day so they could close early and be with their families that evening. I was scheduled for 7:45AM. The following day both the chemo lab and the radiation lab were closed and treatments were cancelled so we could all be with our families on Christmas Day. It was a precious time for all of my family to be able to celebrate with our Mother and Dad who were getting on up in age. Both of them were mobile, their minds were clear as a bell and they were able to stay at home without having anyone helping them. My Mother was a good cook, but we all brought food so that she would not have so much to do. Richard's Mother had arthritis, which was giving her a lot of pain in her back and legs; but she was still able to stay at home, and she was a good cook, too, which was a real blessing. We offered to have Christmas Eve at our house; but she said as long as she was able, she wanted to have it at her house, so that is what we did. Everyone brought food there, too. Cooking and eating were a big part of all of our celebrations.

The day after Christmas, which was on Thursday, it was back to the chemo lab at 8:45 AM. That week I was not scheduled for radiation until 4:30 PM because the lab was trying to shuffle appointments to get everyone in who had missed treatments during the holiday. The next week we had to shuffle schedules once again because of the New Year holiday. December 31st was on Tuesday, so radiation treatments were cancelled for New Year's Eve and

New Year's Day, and the chemo lab would also be closed that day. So, after completing my fourth chemo treatment on Thursday and my seventeenth radiation treatment on Monday December 30th, I wouldn't have any treatments until NEXT YEAR! Soon it would be a new year and a new beginning, and I was anxiously anticipating both.

CHAPTER EIGHT

THE MONTH OF JANUARY

HAPPY NEW YEAR!

January. If you just think about that word, it brings visions of freezing temperatures, freezing rain and ice and snow, but when you say "New Year," now that's a word that you can really get excited about! I had high hopes for this New Year and its promises of better days and better health. We had a wonderful Christmas with our usual family gatherings, and Shelly stayed over with us from Monday until Thursday, which was a real blessing. She had been very supportive, even with her busy teaching and coaching schedule. I was thankful for this new day and for this new year. Most of all I was encouraged each day with the knowledge that I was being lifted up in prayer by loving and caring people. I know God hears the prayers of the righteous. I prayed God's blessings on each of them every day.

I was just counting down the days until all of my treatments would be completed, after which I would be scheduled for another CT Scan. With the removal of the cancer and finally being able to get clear margins, I was considered pathologically cancer free. The treatments that I was undergoing were standard procedure for prevention of this highly recurrent cancer. I still had to remind myself to take one day at a time and that each day is a gift from God. I am mindful that in God's good keeping all is well.

As I began my tenth month of treatment and looked back on all I had been through and considered how God and the prayers of the people had sustained me, I was humbled. I was still sending out updates to everyone to let them know about my progress and my experiences. I know that in the future when I hear of someone who is going through cancer treatment, it will have a whole new meaning for me and, I am sure, also for everyone who was receiving my progress reports. I continued to be overwhelmed and humbled by the outpouring of compassion that I received in so many ways and from so many people. My heart has been touched by the expressions of love and I have been forever changed in a way that I hope will bring glory to God as I endeavor to witness to His sustaining power in all circumstances.

TREATMENTS INTERUPTED

On Thursday, January 2nd, I was scheduled for both a chemo treatment and a radiation treatment to make up for missing them on the New Year holiday. The chemo was at 8:45 AM and the radiation was at 11:30 AM, so we had to make two trips that day. I was still tolerating the treatments fairly well. I had not had the drop in blood counts as before.

On Wednesday January 8th, I finished my sixth chemo treatment, which put me at the halfway mark for completion of these treatments, and I had my twenty-second radiation treatment. Everything was going along just fine and I was really anticipating having all of this behind me. My energy level was still low, but I was doing OK.

Then, on Wednesday, January 15th, things started to change. We arrived at the chemo lab for my seventh chemo treatment, and I had the usual needle-puncture for the blood work to be done. My oncologist called me into her office and went over the results of the blood test, and unfortunately my counts were too low to be able to take the treatment today. I received a procrit shot to boost my counts and was rescheduled for the next Wednesday. This was so very disappointing. But if that wasn't enough, when we got to the radiation lab and my radiation oncologist examined me, she said that the burns were getting so bad that we might have to stop the radiation and the chemo. The reason the burns were so bad is that apparently the chemo had intensified the effects of the radiation. I told her about my blood counts being low and that my regularly scheduled chemo treatment had already been cancelled that day. I also told her that I was making it OK with the burns and I asked her what the determining factor would be that would result in stopping the radiation treatments. I really wanted to continue if at all possible in order to finish them and get them behind me. She said that the determining factor would be when the second layer of skin falls off, we would definitely have to stop. Well! Now that she had explained it to me, I would have no problem with stopping the treatments for a while. So, that is what we decided to do, because in addition to the burns and my blood counts being too low, she detected that I also had acquired a staff infection in the area of the radiation burn. It was a real bummer day. I could feel the discouragement sweep over me. It was almost overwhelming.

I was placed on antibiotics to treat the staff infection. I only missed five radiation treatments before I was able to resume the schedule. I returned to the chemo lab on Wednesday, January 22nd, hoping that I would be able to continue with the treatment; but when my oncologist examined me, she asked me if I was having any difficulty breathing or if I had been coughing. I told her that I had a slight cold and cough. She said that my lungs really sounded bad. She thought that I might have pneumonia. She ordered a lung x-ray right away. The treatment was cancelled until the results of the x-ray could be read. We went home to wait to hear the results. The next day we reported to the radiation lab to see if it would be possible to resume the radiation treatments. The burns were definitely improving, so I was allowed to take the treatment that day. During the examination before the treatment, the radiology oncologist seemed very concerned about one large blister that had popped up below the burn area. It was caused by the staff infection. She was almost distraught over the fact that it was going to leave a scar. I didn't understand her concern. I thought to myself, "Have you seen the scar left up here where my breast used to be? Who cares about a little scar from a blister?" When we arrived home we had a message about the lung x-ray and it was good news! No pneumonia; but the doctor still wanted to wait another week before resuming the treatments. I was again placed on antibiotics as a precaution.

AT THE CROSS, AT THE CROSS
WHERE I FIRST SAW THE LIGHT!

As you might imagine, I was beginning to feel very discouraged. My energy level was really down then. My one sustaining thought was that we were continually being lifted in prayer by so many friends, and that somehow we would get through all of this.

On Friday, January 24th, I returned to the radiation lab for my twenty-seventh treatment. When I was on the table taking the treatment, I realized that I was surrounded by some of the most elaborate and sophisticated technology equipment available; but as I looked up at the ceiling I noticed that someone had hand carved a very primitive cross shape in one of the ceiling tiles directly above the table, and that there were red lights shining through the carving. The lights were positioned at the top of the cross and on both sides of the cross bar. All of a sudden the carving and the red lights reminded me of the cross and the suffering that Jesus had endured. I asked the radiation technician why the cross was carved in the ceiling and what was the purpose of the red lights? He said the opening was to allow the red laser lights to shine through and down on the patient. These lights were positioned there to aid them in determining where the radiation should be directed. As I lay there on the table, with my arm in the usual uncomfortable position (now due to the burns more than the surgery) I was able to focus on the cross. It really put my pain in a whole new and different perspective. This thought gave me strength and courage and really lifted the burden that was hanging over my heart. I had been sustained through all of my treatments up until now, and I knew that I would be sustained until they were completed.

WHY ME LORD?

Even though I was feeling better, on the way home from this treatment I began to question why all of this was happening to me. At some point in our lives we have all said that: "Why me Lord?" This reminded me of a poem that I had written on Easter morning in 1985. It had been almost one year since our precious daughter, Lynn, had been killed in an automobile accident while on her way home from school. Just before going to church on that Easter morning, I sat down and in just a very short time I had written this poem that just seemed to flow out of my thoughts onto the paper. I want to share it with others in the hope that it will help someone who might find themselves sometimes asking, "Why me Lord?" I know it has been a comfort to me throughout these many years since that day.

> Sometimes we say "Why me Lord?
> How could this happen to me?
> I've always trusted in your name
> Why didn't you intervene?
>
> Then I remembered long ago
> A life once lived to show
> What really is important
> In this life on earth below

When you came to live here
You had no easy way
The very night that you were born
Was in a manger filled with hay

We know your earthly father
Must have died when you were young
For there was no mention of him
When from that cross you were hung

And when I think of that cross
On Calvary's hill that day
I wonder why ten thousand angels
Didn't come and take you away

You shouldn't have had to suffer
You're the Father's only Son
Why didn't God come and save YOU?
That's what He could have done

But God loves us all very much
And He wanted us to see
That we can still trust in Him
Even hanging from a tree

Faith in God is what we need
To make it through our trials
And we have the great example
Of our Father's only child

Jesus knew what lay in store
In heaven up above
He knew He'd see His Father's face
And all of those he loves

When I miss my Lynn
Who died at Sweet Sixteen
I often wonder why my Lord
Didn't come and intervene

But I will always trust Him
For I know what is in store
I have a hope of being with Lynn
At Easter time once more

—Nina Anderson 1985

By Thursday, January 30th, I was taking my thirty-second radiation treatment. I was thinking, "only three more to go". When I finished, the radiologist called me into her office to let me know that I would be scheduled for my last treatment the next day. This would be what is called a booster treatment, which would be more intense than all of the others. She called it the Super Dose. I was so excited to be planning for my "last radiation treatment". I was beginning to wonder if I was ever going to get to say those words. But here we were. I was just so overwhelmed by the reality of it all. So, on the last day of January, I reported to the radiation lab for the last time for my very last radiation treatment! I felt such relief! Once again, it was like a burden had been lifted. Thanks be to God and praise His Holy name!

I praised God for sustaining not only me, but Richard and Shelly as well. They had been so great through all of this, always encouraging me and being there with me. There had been times when I had thought about not continuing the treatments, especially when we had to stop; but somehow, when I needed the courage to overcome the fears, God provided it along with a peace about the situation. I believe all of this was a direct result of the prayers offered on my behalf; and I am exceedingly grateful to God for His mercy and grace given to each one of us.

CHAPTER NINE

THE SAGA CONTINUES

SOME DAYS ARE DIAMOND

I sure was glad to see February. This would be the beginning of my eleventh month of treatment. We certainly experienced enough setbacks during the previous month. The completion of the radiation treatments was the highlight of the year so far. I only had five more chemo treatments to go. Five more weeks—that sounded so good.

All of the remaining chemo treatments were uneventful, and I was so very thankful for that. As each week passed, so did another treatment. By Wednesday, March 5th, I was actually reporting to the chemo lab for my last chemo! It was very difficult to keep from dancing my way into the lab. This would certainly qualify for a diamond day and one in which to celebrate! Some have warned me that when the treatments are finally over some patients sink into a depression because there is nothing else to do to fight the cancer. But I didn't think that would ever happen to me. I was so joyful to finally have all of this behind me. Now, hopefully, we could get back to somewhat of a normal life and a normal schedule. PRAISE THE LORD!

I am truly thankful for chemo, but I am also thankful to be finished with it. In all, I had twenty chemo treatments, three major surgeries, thirty-three radiation treatments, a staff infection and an allergic reaction to antibiotics. I was scheduled for a CBC on Friday, March 7th, and the first of my weekly CA 27-29 tumor marker tests, which can help in the detection of any presence of breast cancer. It is somewhat like the PSA test, which is used to help in the detection of prostate cancer in men. Everyone who has had breast cancer has a CA 27-29 tumor marker range which would normally be between 0-38. So, we would be checking this each week for a while. By the last week in March, with all of my tumor marker test results being in the normal range, my oncologist extended the testing period to one month. This was another diamond day for me!!

SURVIVORSHIP

When April 5th rolled around, it marked my one year anniversary of my diagnosis of malignant Inflammatory Breast Cancer. I tried to find out if I should count being a survivor from the date of my diagnosis or from the date of my last treatment, but so far I haven't been able to get a definite answer. Apparently everybody has their own opinion. So, if it is from the time of the last treatment, I was celebrating my one-month survivorship; but if it was from the time of my diagnosis, I was celebrating my one-year survivorship. Whichever it was, I was on a roll!

Even though it had been one month since my last treatment, I was still dealing with fatigue. My oncologist told me that in time this would diminish. Also, I was left with a few reminders of my treatments. I had numbness in my hands and feet (neuropathy) caused by the chemotherapy. I was told that in time this would also disappear, so I was looking forward to that. I was also looking forward to a full head of hair. It seemed that it was growing very slowly, but at least it was growing back.

I was sitting at my desk preparing an update to send to all my family, friends and prayer warriors to let them know how I was doing. I looked out of my window in my office and there was a bumble bee hovering there. I couldn't help thinking back to that Friday in April of the previous year, when I sat in another chair taking my first chemo treatment and watched the bumble bees flying outside the window. I remembered the sweet revelation that God had given me through this fuzzy, furry, fat little fellow. On that day I had remembered reading somewhere that, according to the laws of aerodynamics, bumblebees can't fly. It's impossible! But there they were, leaping over tall buildings, sometimes at the speed of bullets; and I suddenly realized that if bumblebees can fly, then anything is possible with God as our Creator. What a beautiful revelation!

I felt like I had come full-circle, because once again God used the bumble bee to remind me that it was God who had sustained me throughout the last twelve months and had continued to fill me with hope, just as He did on that very first day. I have learned that each day is a gift and to trust in God more and more as each day passes.

The bumble bees were flying, and I was cancer free. Will miracles never cease? I praised the God who forgives our iniquities and heals our diseases (Psalm 103), and thanked Him for all He had done for me. Since Inflammatory Breast Cancer is so highly recurrent, my oncologist asked me to remain vigilant and observant, and to report anything that might indicate a recurrence or metastasis. I was scheduled to see her once a month for blood chemistry testing, which was to continue for at least one year. I was also scheduled for a CT Scan on Monday, May 12th. This would be my first scan since completing all of my treatments. The following is an excerpt from the update which I sent out to my family, friends and prayer warriors regarding the results of this scan.

Dear Family, Friends and Prayer Warriors!

I have great news to report! I went for a CT Scan last Monday and except for scarring in my right lung, I have an all clear report! Praise the Lord! Hallelujah! And to God be the Glory! I have been walking on a cloud since we got the news and wanted to share it with you so that you could rejoice with us! I am eternally grateful for all of your prayers and your expressions of support throughout my 400+ day ordeal. I still need for you to remember me and my family in the days ahead as we remain vigilant against the recurrence of this cancer.

There were some concerns listed in the CT Scan report regarding a new "patch" that showed up in my right lung and that a PET Scan might be in order. However, both my oncologist and her physician assistant gave the opinion that it was radiation scarring, but just to be on the safe side, they sent it to my radiation oncologist who confirmed their opinion. So we had three people who are experts/specialists in this area that agreed that it was radiation scarring! I am scheduled for another CT Scan in two to three months.

I am feeling better everyday. The only pills I am taking are vitamins, which by the way I was not allowed to take during my long treatment process. This was an area that I had some conflict about but I decided to follow the advice of my oncologist. I hope that more research can be done in the future to support the use of supplements during chemo, surgery and radiation, which will scientifically prove that it is beneficial. Right now there is not enough data to support this and there is some concern that the anti-oxidants in the supplements would counteract the effects of the treatments.

I am left with a few reminders of my treatments, one of which is numbness in the bottom of my feet. They say this may go away or it may not. Also, I still experience some pain and sensitivity in the incision/radiation area and under my right arm and my veins are not as good as they use to be. I had twenty chemo treatments without a port. We are hopeful that all of this will improve with time. As they say, "Time heals all wounds".

Once again, thank you for your prayers and your care and concern during this time. Sometimes just knowing that you all were praying for me was all that kept me going.

May God continue to bless you as He blesses us!

I was scheduled to continue seeing my oncologist on a regular monthly basis for one year. However, after the third month, I was doing so well that she extended the time between my visits to every two months. We did that for two months and she extended the visits to every three months. I was really beginning to feel like all of this was behind me. When I finally reached the twenty-four month anniversary since my last treatment, my oncologist informed me that for Inflammatory Breast Cancer, which was so aggressive, this was like the five-year mark for other breast cancers. I was overjoyed to hear this wonderful news. The Physician's Assistant who was also there that day was very excited and happy for me. We both remembered what the doctor at the M. D. Anderson Cancer Center had told me on my fifty-sixth birthday. She said that it was almost 100% certain that the cancer would come back! This just goes to show that everyone is different when it comes to the statistics of cancer.

I would still have some anxious times during the next few years but as the bumble bee still reminds me, ALL THINGS ARE POSSIBLE WITH GOD AS OUR CREATOR!

> "I love the Lord because he hears my prayers and answers them. Because he bends down and listens, I will pray as long as I breathe! Death stared me in the face—I was frightened and sad. Then I cried, "Lord, save me!" How kind he is! How good he is! So merciful, this God of ours! The Lord protects the simple and the childlike; I was facing death and then he saved me. Now, I can relax. For the Lord has done this wonderful miracle for me. He has saved me from death, my eyes from tears, and my feet from stumbling. I shall live! Yes, in his presence—here on earth!"—Psalms 116:1-9, *The Living Bible.*

TIME LINE—INFLAMMATORY BREAST CANCER

CHAPTER ONE—APRIL, 2002

April 5, 2002	Fri	Mammogram
April 10, 2002	Wed	Appt. with surgeon and biopsy
April 15, 2002	Mon	Test Results—Malignant, Inflammatory Breast Cancer,
April 16, 2002	Tue	Appointment with oncologist Scheduled pre chemotherapy testing Scheduled 1st chemotherapy treatment for 4/19/02
April 17, 2002	Thur	9:00 AM Injection for Bone Scan, 12:00 PM Bone Scan and Brain Scan
April 18, 2002	Thur	CT Scan with pre-medication for Iodine Alergy, Echo Cardiogram Purchased a wig
April 19, 2002	Fri	8:00 AM Appt. for Second Opinion 10:30 AM Ordered Her-2-neu and ER/PR tests on tissue from biopsy 11:00-4:30 PM Results of CT Scans and Tests 1st chemotherapy treatment, Adriamycin/Cytoxan(A/C)

April 22, 2002   Mon.   Decided to follow second opinion oncologist
                              Requested all records be sent to new oncologist

April 24-28, 2002   Wed   Mini-Vacation to Panama City Beach

CHAPTER TWO—MAY, 2002

May 1, 2002   Wed   10th day after chemo, blood test (CBC) to check
                              blood cell counts
May 2, 2002   Thur   Hair starts falling out
May 3, 2002   Fri   CBC to re-check blood cell counts
                              Celebrated my Dad's 86th birthday
May 5, 2002   Sun   Celebrated Shelly's 29th birthday
May 8, 2002   Wed.   2nd A/C chemotherapy treatment.
May 10, 2002   Fri   Procrit Shot to help boost red blood cells
                              Started daily self injections of Leukine to help
                              boost white blood cells
May 12, 2002   Sun   Celebrated Mother's Day
                              Ordered New Wig
May 17, 2002   Fri   10th day CBC
May 23, 2002   Thur   CBC to re-check blood cell counts
May 25, 2002   Sat   Lynn's death date remembered—It has been 18
                              years
May 29, 2002   Wed   3rd A/C chemotherapy treatment
May 31, 2002   Fri   Procrit Shot and start Leukine self injections again

CHAPTER THREE-SUMMER, 2002

June 5, 2002   Wed   10th day CBC to check blood cell counts
June 7, 2002   Fri   CBC to recheck blood cell counts—Another
                              Procrit Shot
                              Appointment with surgeon.
                              Sonogram to check progress of reduction of tumor
                              Unable to get imaging of illusive tumor

June 12, 2002   Wed   CBC to re-check blood cell counts
                              Cell counts too low—Procrit shot and continue
                              with Leukine shots
June 16, 2002   Sun   Celebrated Father's Day

June 17, 2002	Mon	CBC to re-check blood cell counts—continue Leukine
June 18, 2002	Tue	Annual Pap Test and Physical Exam
June 19, 2002	Wed.	CANCELLED chemotherapy treatment. Counts were still too low.
June 19, 2002	Wed	Reaction to antibiotic
June 20, 2002	Thur	New antibiotic prescribed
June 24, 2002	Mon	CBC-Counts are improving
June 26, 2002	Wed.	4th A/C chemotherapy treatment. Reported that Leukine shots were making me feel very bad.
June 28, 2002	Fri	CBC to check blood cell counts Procrit shot and changed from Leukine to Neulasta for boosting white blood cells.
July 4th, 2002	Thur	Celebrated 4th of July Missed Annual Antique Steam Powered Tractor Parade
July 5, 2002	Fri	CBC to check blood cell counts. Procrit shot
July 10, 200	Wed	CBC to re-check blood cell counts. Another Procrit shot
July 12, 2002	Fri	CT Scan to recheck spots on liver from April Scans
July 16, 2002	Tue	Results from CT Scan and Start pre-meds for chemotherapy treatment of Taxotere
July 17, 2002	Wed	5th chemotherapy treatment—1st Taxotere
July 18, 2002	Thur	Neulasta shot and Procrit shot
July 19-21,2002	Fri.	Spent the weekend at Walt Allen's house in Cashiers, NC.
July 20, 2002	Sat	Having second thoughts
July 26, 2002	Fri	CBC to check blood cell counts. Procrit Shot
August 7, 2002	Wed.	6th chemotherapy treatment—2nd Taxotere
August 9, 2002	Fri	Neulasta shot and Procrit shot
August 16, 2002	Fri	CBC to check blood cell counts
August 20, 2002	Tue	Eye Exam—a floater appeared in right eye.
August 28, 2002	Wed	7th chemo treatment—3rd Taxotere
August 30, 2002	Fri	Neulasta shot. Procrit Shot

CHAPTER FOUR—SEPTEMBER, 2002

September 4, 2002	Wed	Consultation for surgery. Modified Radical Mastectomy.
September 6, 2002	Fri	CBC to check blood cell counts
September 14, 2002	Sat.	Lynn's 35th birthday remembered.
September 18, 200	Wed.	8th and last chemotherapy treatment before surgery—4th Taxotere
September 20, 2002	Fri	Neulasta shot. Procrit Shot. Celebrated Richard's 57th birthday.
September 25, 2002	Wed.	Celebrated our 37th wedding anniversary
September 27, 2002	Fri	CBC to check blood cell counts. OK No Shots

CHAPTER FIVE—OCTOBER, 2002

October 3, 2002	Thur	Telephone assessment for surgery.
October 4, 2002	Fri	Consultation with Plastic Surgeon
October 14, 2002	Mon	Dental Appointment
October 17, 2002	Thur	Surgery 1:00 PM Northside Hospital.
October 18, 2002	Fri.	Pathology Report—Did not get clean margins Discussed options. Home from hospital
October 23, 2002	Wed	Post Operative check-up with surgeon. Scheduled a biopsy for October 30.
October 24, 2002	Thur	Started taking the hormone, Femara, as a continuation of treatment for cancer.
October 29, 2002	Tue	Pre-op consultation with plastic surgeon for partial reconstruction
October 30, 2002	Wed	Biopsy to try and determine cancer margins.
October 31, 2002	Thur	Physical therapy for right arm after surgery.

CHAPTER SIX—NOVEMBER, 2002

November 1, 2002	Fri	Appointment with a radiology oncologist Scheduled 35 radiation treatments
November 2-6, 2002	Sat	Mini vacation to Panama City Beach. A time for reflection and planning what next.

November 8, 2002	Fri	Physical therapy
November 10, 2002	Sun	Drive to MD Anderson Cancer Center in Orlando, FL to get second opinion on course of action on remaining cancer.
November 11, 2002	Mon	Appointment with a doctor at 8:30AM Celebrated my 56th Birthday in Orlando
November 13, 2002	Wed.	1:00 PM Re-excision Partial reconstruction by plastic surgeon to close incision
Noverber 19, 2002	Tues	10:45 follow up visit to plastic surgeon Lunch. 1:15 follow up visit with surgeon. Hematoma discovered during visit 6:00 PM Emergency surgery to stop bleeding.
November 20, 2002	Wed	Released from hospital. Follow up appointment with oncologist Discussed Femara and ER/PR test reading Requested new radiologist closer home
November 25, 2002	Mon	3:00 PM follow up visit with surgeon Picked up mammogram x-rays for radiology oncologist
November 26, 2002	Tue	8:30 AM CT Scan with pre medication and contrast 1:00 PM Consultation with radiology oncologist Brought mammograms and CT Scans.
November 28, 2002	Thu	Celebrated Thanksgiving Day

CHAPTER SEVEN—DECEMBER, 2002

December 2, 2002	Mon	Physical Therapy after 2nd and 3rd surgeries
December 4, 2002	Wed.	1st of twelve chemotherapy treatments with Taxol
December 5, 2002	Thur	1st of thirty-five radiation treatments
December 6, 2002	Fri	2nd radiation treatment
December 9, 2002	Mon	3rd radiation treatment

December 10, 2002 Tues   4th radiation treatment
December 11, 2002 Wed   9:00 AM 2nd chemotherapytreatment
                           12:00 Christmas Lunch with my company
                           4:30 PM 5th radiation treatment
December 12, 2002 Thur   6th radiation treatment
December 13, 2002 Fri   7th radiation treatment
December 16, 2002 Mon   1:00 PM Physical Thereapy 4:30 PM 8th
                           radiation treatment
December 17, 2002 Tue   9th radiation treatment
December 18, 2002 Wed.   8:15 AM 3rd chemotherapy treatment
                           4:30 PM 10th radiation treatment
December 19, 2002 Thur   11th radiation treatment
December 20, 2002 Fri   12th radiation treatment
December 23, 2002 Mon   10:30 AM Physical Therapy
                           4:30 PM 13th radiation treatment
December 24, 2002 Tue   7:45 AM 14th radiation treatment
                           Celebrated Christmas Eve
December 25, 2002 Wed   Celebrated Christmas Day—NO TREATMENTS
December 26, 2002 Thur   8:45 AM 4th chemotherapy treatment
                           4:30PM 15th radiation treatment
December 27, 2002 Fri   16th radiation treatment
December 30, 2002 Mon   17th radiation treatment (half way there)
December 31, 2002 Tue   Celebrated New Year's Eve NO TREATMENT

CHAPTER EIGHT—JANUARY, 2003

January 1, 2003   Wed   Celebrated New Year's Day NO TREATMENT
January 2, 2003   Thur   8:45 AM 5th chemotherapy treatment
                           11:30 AM 18th radiation treatment

January 3, 2003   Fri   19th radiation treatment
January 6, 2003   Mon   20th radiation treatment
January 7, 2003   Tue   21st radiation treatment
January 8, 2003   Wed   8:45 AM 6th chemotherapy treatment (half way there)
                           11:30 AM 22nd radiation treatment

January 9, 2003   Thur   23rd radiation treatment
January 10, 2003   Fri   24th radiation treatment
January 13, 2003   Mon   25th radiation treatment
January 14, 2003   Tue   26th radiation treatment

January 15, 2003	Wed	8:45 AM Blood counts too low
		NO CHEMOTHERAPY TREATMENT
		11:30 AM radiation burns very bad and Staff Infection
		NO RADIATION TREATMENT
January 16, 2003	Thur	NO RADIATION TREATMENT
January 17, 2003	Fri	NO RADIATION TREATMENT
January 20, 2003	Mon	NO RADIATION TREATMENT
January 21, 2003	Tue	NO RADIATION TREATMENT
January 22, 2003	Wed	NO CHEMOTHERAPY AND NO RADIATION
January 23, 2003	Thur	Radiation resumed. 27th radiation treatment
January 24, 2003	Fri	28th radiation treatment
January 27, 2003	Mon	29th radiation treatment
January 28, 2003	Tue	30th radiation treatment
January 29, 2003	Wed	8:45 AM 7th chemotherapy treatment
		11:30 AM 31st radiation treatment
January 30, 2003	Thur	32nd radiation treatment
January 31, 2003	Fri	33rd radiation treatment—Super Dose and last treatment

CHAPTER NINE—THE SAGA CONTINUES

February 5, 2003	Wed	8th chemotherapy treatment
February 12, 2003	Wed	9th chemotherapy treatment—Procrit Shot
February 19, 2003	Wed	10th chemotherapy treatment
February 26, 2003	Wed	11th chemotherapy treatment
March 5, 2003	Wed	12th and FINAL chemotherapy treatment!!!!!
		Follow up with Radiology Oncologist
March 7, 2003	Fri	CBC and CA 27-29 Tumor Marker tests
March 19, 2003	Wed.	CBC and CA 27-29 Tumor Marker tests
March 24, 2003	Mon	CBC and CA 27-29 Tumor Marker tests
		Wait One Month to come back for next tumor marker test!
April 30, 2003	Wed	CBC and CA 27-29 Tumor Marker tests

The saga continues to this day . . . .

REFERENCES

1   I used the most up-to-date information on Inflammatory Breast Cancer at the time of the completion of this book which was July 31, 2007. The article was written by Dr. Jeff Patton of Tennessee Oncology and was taken from the National Breast Cancer Foundation, Inc. website—Breast Cancer Signs & Symptoms—Inflammatory Breast Cancer.

www.ingramcontent.com/pod-product-compliance
Lightning Source LLC
Chambersburg PA
CBHW031241280526
45784CB00004B/1673